Dr. Mik
A

DR MIKE SMITH is an ⌐   ⌐   ⌐ Health
Medicine and President o.   ⌐₌₌ᵤₒᵤᵢₐtion of Broadcasting
Doctors. He was the Chief Medical Officer of the Family
Planning Association 1970–75 and their Honorary Medical
Adviser 1975–90. He is an elected member of the FPA's
National Executive Committee and a member of the
advisory panel of both the National Food Safety Advisory
Centre and the British Association of Continence Care. For
many years he has been a 'resident' expert guest on BBC2's
Jimmy Young Programme, LBC's Nightline and the medical
columnist/editor for Woman's Own. Between 1980 and
1984 he presented BBC1's health series 'Looking Good,
Feeling Fit' and from 1988–90 he was the expert guest on
SKY TV's 'Sky by Day'. In April 1991, he was voted the TV
and Radio Doctors' 'Experts' Expert' in the Observer
magazine's series.

His other books include *Birth Control*, *How to Save Your
Child's Life*, *A New Dictionary of Symptoms* and *Dr Mike Smith's
Handbook of Over-the-Counter Medicines*.

Also in *Dr Mike Smith's Postbag* series:

Stress

Back-Pain

H.R.T.

DR MIKE SMITH'S

POSTBAG

ARTHRITIS

WITH SHARRON KERR

KYLE CATHIE LIMITED

First published 1993 by
Kyle Cathie Limited
3 Vincent Square
London SW1P 2LX

ISBN 1 85626 085 2

A CIP catalogue record for this title
is available from the British Library

Typeset by DP Photosetting, Aylesbury, Bucks
Printed and bound in Great Britain by
Butler & Tanner Ltd, Frome and London

CONTENTS

Introduction   1

The Common Forms of Arthritis   3
  Osteoarthritis   5
  Rheumatoid Arthritis   10
  Ankylosing Spondylitis   18
  Psoriasis and Arthritis   24
  Colitis, Crohn's Disease and Arthritis   28
  Gout   33
  Systemic Lupus Erythematosus (SLE)   38

Arthritis and Treatment   45
  When to Seek Help and What to Say   46
  Drugs   49
  Surgery   51
  Physiotherapy   55
  Occupational Therapy   60

Self-help Treatment   68
  Arthritis, Diet, Supplements and Lucky Charms   70
  Exercise – and Rest   82
  Relaxation Techniques   84
  Positive Thinking   85

Complementary or Alternative Treatments   93
  Acupuncture   93
  Homeopathy   96
  Osteopathy   97
  Chiropractic   98

Useful Addresses   99
Index   104

INTRODUCTION

I'm sure most people will know someone who suffers from arthritis, be it only mildly or much more severely. Yet, I'm also certain that not everyone understands exactly what arthritis is – if the letters I receive in my postbag are anything to go by.

First, I'd like to clear up one of the questions I'm constantly asked: 'What's the difference between rheumatism and arthritis?' Joint problems can often affect nearby bone, muscles and ligaments and the general term 'rheumatism' may then be used to describe the resulting aches and pains. These can, of course, also occur unrelated to arthritis – for example, due to muscle strain – and are then usually temporary. So, 'rheumatism' is the general term for referring to any sort of aching pain in the bones, muscles or joints, and 'arthritis' the general term for inflammation, disease of, or damage to a joint. It's used to describe any type of joint disease, even when there is no inflammation involved. So, contrary to common belief, arthritis isn't just a single rheumatic disease; there are, in fact, more than two hundred kinds of rheumatic disease, some extremely unusual and others very common.

It's thought that in any one year, as many as 20 million people could be suffering from some form of rheumatic disease. More than £150 million is spent on prescription drugs to relieve arthritis and an amazing 88 million working days are lost each year because of the condition. One report even suggests that arthritis costs Britain £1200 million annually in medical bills and loss of earnings.

As there is a tremendous range of arthritic conditions, I'll deal here with some of the most widespread. This book is intended as a guide to understanding arthritis not as a substitute for medical consultation and diagnosis. I hope it will answer some of your unasked questions – questions some of you might have written to me about – as well as giving you practical advice and pointers about where to go for further help.

THE COMMON FORMS OF ARTHRITIS

Arthritis refers to something much more than an aching pain, and being told you have it could mean one of a large number of different things. There are many, many types of arthritis, from osteoarthritis through to reactive arthritis – which can be a relatively shortlived type of inflammation of the joints after a viral infection such as glandular fever or German measles (rubella arthritis). Reactive arthritis also covers Reiter's syndrome, which involves conjunctivitis, urethritis (inflammation of the urethra), mouth ulcers, rashes and arthritis, and follows a trigger urogenital or bowel infection.

An example of a rare form of arthritis is polyarteritis nodosa, which causes patches of inflammation in the walls of small- and medium-sized arteries. The restriction of movement this causes when not treated can lead to local arthritis.

On top of this, carpal tunnel syndrome, which involves inflammation of the lining of the carpal tunnel in the wrist, has early-morning symptoms very similar to arthritis, such as pins and needles, tingling, stiffness or pain, and this often causes confusion in diagnosis.

One sufferer told me she has a very simple analogy to explain arthritis: ice cream – the term describes the substance but just look at the different combinations of flavours.

It's true that while some people are hardly even aware they have arthritis and in all honesty feel it makes little difference to their lives, others find everyday life an uphill struggle. In its most severe forms arthritis can be so debilitating that even the most mundane task gives rise to frustration. Just wringing out a dishcloth can become impossible; using a knife and fork can be a trial.

And if, at this point, your mind is filled with typical images of an arthritis sufferer as an old person with twisted, gnarled hands, hardly able to move and hunched over a walking stick, *think again.* In complete contrast to this popular image, arthritis really isn't the scourge of just the elderly.

True, arthritis is more widespread in the older community, particularly osteoarthritis, which is its most common form. This tends to affect people in middle and later life and can run in families. It is aggravated by the general wear and tear of the ageing process, which can cause changes in the body's joints. Nearly half of all people over the age of sixty-five have some form of arthritis, but people of all ages, even children, can suffer from its various forms.

You may be surprised to learn that as many as one in every twenty sixteen- to forty-four-year-olds suffers from arthritis. Yet people still express surprise when they discover that a friend or relative in his or her twenties or thirties has one of its forms. Almost every younger arthritis sufferer I've spoken to has repeated this fact.

The sad thing is that arthritis affects some 15,000 children in the UK. It frequently begins between the ages of one and four and is generally referred to as juvenile arthritis or juvenile chronic arthritis, although just to add to the complicated picture there are several different types of childhood arthritis (but I am not going to deal with them in detail. They would warrant a whole book to themselves). There is one positive aspect about juvenile arthritis and that is the outlook is often good. Many children do improve with the excellent medical care available these days. For adults, and despite the millions of people suffering from the disease at any given time, the outlook is often not quite as good.

There is still no cure for arthritis, the causes are not fully understood and there's no way of telling who will develop it and who will not. Even the experts themselves can't agree. For example, they're divided when it comes to pinpointing climate as a factor in the development of the disease. Arthritis is a worldwide problem in hot or cold climates, although severer forms of rheumatoid arthritis certainly seem to occur more frequently in northern Europe. There's also a great deal of argument over the cause and effect of diet in relation to arthritis (so much so that I'll be devoting a section of this book specifically to the subject, see pages 70–81) despite some sufferers' insistence that certain food aggravates their symptoms. And as to the precise role of bacteria in the disease, some experts argue that, despite isolated incidents, researchers have failed to consistently find bacteria in the joints of people with rheumatoid arthritis.

Scientists do believe they have identified the gene responsible for arthritis, although it does not itself cause the disease. Some other factor in the environment – possibly a type of virus – is also involved. It seems that people probably develop arthritis because of a combination of different factors rather than one single cause. But so far a cure for the condition is proving elusive and for the moment we can only live in the hope that researchers will one day develop a vaccine to banish this painful and often crippling disease.

OSTEOARTHRITIS

Osteoarthritis, also called osteoarthrosis or degenerative joint disease, is as I've already mentioned the most common form of arthritis throughout the world. It is estimated that there are around 5 million sufferers in this country alone.

Don't listen to old wives' tales that imply the more you use your joints the more likely you are to develop arthritis. Over-use of joints doesn't cause osteoarthritis – sportsmen, for instance, aren't any more likely to develop the disease unless their joints are injured. The wear and tear of the ageing process does, however, seem to play a part in *how badly* you develop the disease and that's probably why osteoarthritis is so common among older people.

Osteoarthritis usually affects the over-fifties, and not many people can escape some degree of it in their old age.

But something you soon learn when you talk about arthritis is that there are virtually no hard and fast rules – osteoarthritis can also be evident in people in their teens or twenties.

Val, a sixty-year-old housewife, has experienced the intense pain and stiffness of osteoarthritis for more than forty years. She was diagnosed as having the disease when she was in her teens.

> Officially I've had osteoarthritis since I was seventeen. I first noticed something was wrong when I was in school in my early teens. It started as pains in my legs and I was told it was growing pains.
>
> But I couldn't run the way the other children did, even though I really wanted to. It was as if my body could run but my legs wouldn't let it. I used to ask other girls whether they had growing pains like this but nobody seemed to.
>
> When I was seventeen I saw a doctor about it because I was losing sleep as a result of the pain, and his exact words were, 'God help you, you've got osteoarthritis.' I didn't know what he was talking about. I certainly didn't realise then how much suffering it would cause me for the rest of my life.

The pain and stiffness in Val's knees and ankles gradually became worse in her twenties and by the time she was thirty-two she could walk only with the help of a stick. She used to work in a shop, but when she was forty-five she felt so crippled with arthritis that she had to give it up.

> I'm the type of person who won't give in easily and I will battle to the bitter end but when I was forty-five I had to stop work.
>
> I don't remember the last time I had a good night's sleep. Sitting still is impossible – I have to wriggle around like an eel to find some relief. The pain of osteoarthritis is an aggravating pain that makes you

want to move your legs like an engine all night long, even though it hurts to move them.

The pain and discomfort is much worse when I have been still for a while. So I have to have short walks, even if it means just walking around my living room. And I do that day and night. When I was younger I seemed to be able to cope with the pain better even if I hadn't slept very well the night before.

Arthritis is such an unsociable disease. I find it's very difficult to go out, say, to the theatre or the cinema. I've tried a few times with my husband. But it's impossible for me to sit still for very long.

When I have gone to the theatre we make sure we are there early so that I can sit at the end of a row and stretch my legs. I've even gone to the ladies' toilet to take a painkiller and I've waited there until it has had some effect before going back to my seat.

Val has found that her osteoarthritis goes through bad patches then settles down again. But after each bout her mobility has become slightly worse. During her fifties she also began to be troubled by rheumatoid arthritis in her hands and feet. By the time she was fifty-eight she was forced to have a wheelchair.

I could hardly walk by then. I could manage to make it around the supermarket if my husband drove me there. Just being able to do that made me happy but that was all I could do.

The wheelchair sat in my house for two weeks and I wouldn't even look at it let alone go in it. Finally my husband, Howard, told me that he was going to take me out in it and I had to go.

I'll never forget how I felt. I was wearing a mac and I pulled the hood right up to try to hide my face as there were tears streaming down it. I'd fought against arthritis all my life. Now I felt as if this was it. My independence had totally gone. It was a terrible feeling.

By now the pain and swelling caused by fluid gathering in Val's knees was so intense it was almost unbearable no matter which painkillers she was prescribed. She was offered a complete knee replacement on her right leg – an offer she gladly accepted. Five months of physiotherapy followed surgery.

> When the specialist saw the x-ray of my knees he was amazed I'd managed to walk a couple of steps. Apparently there was hardly anything left of the joints. He gave me a fifty-fifty chance of success and as I was in a wheelchair I didn't see that I had anything to lose. The mobility is marvellous although I can't walk very far, but I still experience pain. It seems as if I've been in pain all my life.

Although Val's case is extreme, it hits home the point that age and wear and tear are not the prime causes of osteoarthritis. My postbag regularly contains letters from people like Val, challenging the accepted picture of the condition.

The disease causes so much pain because it damages joint surface thus inhibiting the painless and proper use of the joint. When osteoarthritis develops, the protective, shock-absorbing rubbery substance called cartilage, which covers the ends of the bones at the joints to protect them, becomes worn and rough and is almost 'rubbed away'. In places it splits so that the bone underneath thickens and spreads out, enlarging the joint. The disease causes such damage to the surface of the joint that it can't work properly. The bones rub against each other causing pain and stiffness which become worse after keeping still.

Bony outgrowths or spurs – called osteophytes – may develop at the edges of the joints, adding to the gnarled appearance of the sufferer's hands. Knobbly swellings over the finger joints, called Heberden's nodes or Bouchard's nodes, are also common.

Fluid often forms in knees damaged by osteoarthritis, there may be some swelling and tenderness in other affected joints and their surrounding membrane may also become slightly inflamed. As a consequence the joint becomes stiff and painful.

Osteoarthritis tends to involve gradual deterioration and a slow onset of pain and disfigurement as the cartilage is worn away and the bones rub together. The ligaments which allow the joint its full range of natural movement are weakened and the shape of the joint becomes deformed.

Apart from pain and stiffness, symptoms can include tenderness over some joints and 'cracking' noises. Osteoarthritis is not accompanied by general feelings of ill-health, or a high temperature, or loss of appetite, or nausea: pain is its most noticeable feature – dull, persistent pain that becomes more severe when the arthritic joint is moved. Although some sufferers have described it to me as a sharp shooting pain in the joints, it can become constant as the disease worsens – even when you are resting your joints. At its worst, osteoarthritis is very distressing and very disabling; but more often, the symptoms remain mild to moderate and can be effectively relieved. After a couple of years a few sufferers find their condition improves. Most find the disease slowly worsens, then seems to settle down.

Osteoarthritis mainly affects the weight-bearing joints and those in constant use such as knees, hips, spine and fingers. Sometimes the neck and lower back are involved. Shoulders are commonly the last to be affected.

The disease can affect just one joint, when it's referred to as monarticular. But usually a number of joints are affected, although osteoarthritis doesn't travel steadily through the body like rheumatoid arthritis (see page 10).

An injury does make a joint more likely to develop osteoarthritis, when it is referred to as secondary osteoarthritis. Margeret, a sixty-one-year-old housewife, has recently been told she's developed osteoarthritis in her ankle, six months after a fracture. The news came as a great shock.

> Before I broke my ankle I certainly never had any joint pains or stiffness. Six weeks after surgery on my ankle I began physiotherapy twice a week to get the joint moving again. I did stretching exercises, rolling my foot back and forth on a board, moving up and down on my feet. Naturally my ankle was very stiff. I expected that. What I didn't expect was to be told by everyone from my physiotherapist to friends that it was very likely I'd develop arthritis. Their words are turning out to be true. Six months after the accident my ankle is stiffer than ever – I feel as if I have an iron band around it, especially when I've been sitting for a while or when I wake up in the morning.

Some of us are just born with the type of joints that are more likely to develop osteoarthritis – we have a genetic predisposition. Women tend to suffer more than men, especially during the menopause. We don't really know why. Being overweight predisposes to osteoarthritis, too, due to the extra strain, but being overweight doesn't necessarily mean you will develop the disease – quite thin people frequently suffer too!

RHEUMATOID ARTHRITIS

Although not as common as osteoarthritis, rheumatoid arthritis can be far more disabling. An inflammatory disease which makes joints stiff, painful and swollen, it can cause crippling joint damage and the deformities caused are often more severe than those in other forms of arthritis. There are around half a million sufferers from the disease and it remains the most common type of severe arthritis in people below the age of fifty.

Rheumatoid arthritis is a progressive form of arthritis which leads to a gradual deterioration in the affected joints. About a third of patients experience severe disability.

In disease, inflammation most often serves a useful purpose. Its normal function is to protect while healing takes place. Once healing has occurred, the inflammation dies down. This isn't the case with rheumatoid arthritis: the inflammation causes damage itself, and goes on damaging. In fact it can cause so much damage that, for example, the balance between the muscles, tendons and bones in the hand can be destroyed, making movement impossible.

The swelling that develops is a result of a thickening of the synovial membrane, which encases the joint, and the over-production of its usual lubricating fluid. Fluid and cells seep out of the inflamed membrane, disintegrating cartilage. The thickened membrane can also erode the bone ends of the joint as well as their covering cartilage. Surrounding muscles and tendons become swollen and deformed which allows the joint to be pulled out of shape altogether. Unlike osteoarthritis, where the symptoms are often confined to only a few joints, rheumatoid arthritis may affect most of the body's joints.

In rheumatoid arthritis the body's natural defence system overreacts, and the usual mechanism for controlling the immune system seems to fail. Yet it is still uncertain what causes the auto-immunity to behave in this way or even if it behaves in this way because of the arthritis itself. Research has suggested that rheumatoid arthritis could be triggered by a variety of factors, either a viral or bacterial infection which interferes with the body's immune system. This interaction of different factors is probably linked to the sufferer's genetic make-up – some people are just more likely to develop rheumatoid arthritis than others.

So if members of your family have had rheumatoid arthritis, you may be slightly more at risk than someone in a family free of it. But even so, that doesn't mean you're *bound* to suffer from the disease – rheumatoid arthritis is not directly inherited, so please don't worry unduly. In fact, it's really hard to predict just who will develop it. If scientists could discover what sparks off the process they could formulate a treatment for the cause of the disease rather than its symptoms.

While osteoarthritis is most common to older people, rheumatoid arthritis is more likely to affect women in the twenty-to-fifty age group – symptoms very commonly begin around forty. In fact, women are three times more prone to rheumatoid arthritis than men.

Just as in so many forms of the disease, rheumatoid arthritis varies considerably from person to person. However, there is usually a common pattern in that the disease has active and inactive periods – it's likely to be most active in the first few years, before settling down slightly. When it's active, sufferers experience flu-like symptoms with a raised temperature, in addition to swollen, hot, painful joints and stiffness.

Unlike osteoarthritis, where it is usually the large weight-bearing joints which are affected, rheumatoid arthritis tends to strike the smaller joints, for example, in the hands, feet and wrist. These joints are often the most badly affected and are usually the ones that are first to show symptoms of the disease. Sufferers might notice that their hands become stiff, particularly first thing in the morning, and certain activities, like knitting or turning a screwdriver, become slowly more uncomfortable. The fingers can also become swollen and lumpy.

The disease may not progress further, or it can develop in larger joints, as I've said, such as the knees, ankles, elbows, wrists, shoulders and hips. Even other parts of the body, such as the lungs and eyes, can be inflamed. If you have a severe attack of the disease you may need rest in hospital.

I sometimes receive letters from people who have suffered from rheumatoid arthritis for many years and who have recently noticed that their mouth has become very dry and sore and that their eyes also feel dry and uncomfortable. They ask if I know any reason for these symptoms and whether I can suggest anything that might help. If you experience these symptoms you should really consult your doctor and ask him if you could be suffering from Sjogren's syndrome. This is an auto-immune disorder in which the body's immune system turns against itself, attacking the mucous-secreting glands in the body and particularly the salivary and tear-producing ones. Although it is quite common for secretions to dry up a bit as one gets older, a swelling of the salivary glands may also occur. The cause is unknown; it may develop on its own but it is quite often associated with rheumatoid arthritis and other linked conditions such as scleroderma and systemic lupus erythematosus (see page 38).

While only a small percentage of rheumatoid arthritis sufferers develop such conditions, most do complain of pain and loss of strength and mobility in inflamed joints. Stiffness can be worse if a sufferer has been immobile, say after a night's sleep. Morning stiffness is extremely common which is sometimes a result of fluid accumulating in the joints overnight. It's not the stiffness you might feel when you first wake up and which then disappears after a good stretch, but an excessive stiffness that can last for three hours or more and make movement very difficult.

Rheumatoid arthritis is unpredictable but, typically, there are periods of remission when symptoms subside, and these may last months or even years before the next flare-up occurs. The bouts of illness tend to become less and less frequent. According to Arthritis Care, although 30 per cent of sufferers are thought to recover within a few years, about 60 per cent have flare-ups, and in 10 per cent the disease becomes severe and eventually causes disability.

Rheumatoid arthritis sometimes starts quite suddenly but it's more usual for the disease to creep up on you, which is what it did for seventy-one-year-old Isobel. She first noticed symptoms of the disease eight years ago. Five years later it began to affect her life severely and she's now confined to a wheelchair while waiting for operations for shoulder and knee replacements.

One of the many problems faced by a person with

rheumatoid arthritis – along with pain, swelling and stiffness in the affected joints – is wasting of muscles because they have avoided using a painful joint. Sometimes the sufferer notices a weakness in his or her grip. This was what happened to Isobel when the disease first manifested itself.

> I first noticed pain and swollen joints in my fingers. I found holding a knife and putting pressure on it to cut something when I was eating more and more difficult. Then I felt pain in my fingers quite sharply. They'd throb even if I knocked them just slightly.
>
> Then I began to notice a stiffness in the morning which spread from my legs to my knees, arms, neck and now even my jaw. Normally you move without realising you are moving when you first wake up. It wouldn't be a sharp, stabbing pain, more of a dull ache.
>
> I'd have to work out the most painful part (which I still have to do) then gradually move it before starting on the next joint. It could take a while to get out of bed in the morning, which can be difficult if you want to dash to the loo.

Slowly but surely, rheumatoid arthritis has chipped away at Isobel's mobility, although, remarkably, not her spirit. She now has it in both ankles, her right knee is turned inwards and left knee is just starting to become deformed. Both hands are affected and both deformed.

Rheumatoid arthritis causes problems with hands because of the tendons (the tough, fibrous tissue which attaches muscle to bone). Tendons allow the many delicate movements of our hands, and are enclosed in a sheath which is lined by synovial membrane. So when the membrane becomes swollen and inflamed any delicate movement is severely restricted.

For Isobel movement is difficult, not just in her hands. She can't hold a telephone receiver for very long without having to change position, holding her breath while she does it because of the pain.

> I close my eyes and then take a deep breath which I then hold while I move. If I move involuntarily it makes me cry out in pain. For the last three years rheumatoid arthritis has made me severely disabled.
>
> My left thumb is shaped like a letter z. I have a bad right elbow with lots of sharp, stabbing pains which make me cry out. I've been told it's because my shoulder is so bad it's not supporting the bone in my upper arm properly. My left shoulder is painful and stiff. My neck is very stiff and painful in the morning. So is my jaw. And you know I think that's the lot.
>
> I feel fortunate that it's not in my hips because I can get about a little bit. I don't go out very often. I have a wheelchair and I use walking sticks. I cannot grip at all with my fingers. I can just bend them enough to grip a rail at the side of my bed so I can pull myself out. I can't pick up anything small.
>
> As time went on I noticed I couldn't do ordinary things like washing up very well. It's comforting to have my hands in warm water but almost impossible to give anything a good wash. To dry dishes I have to lay a tea cloth on a work surface and place a cup on it. Then I hold the cup with one hand and stroke it dry with a tea towel in the other.
>
> I can't open cupboards. I use a knife as a lever to open my fridge. But I'm determined to carry on doing things.

Although Isobel is coping with courage and resilience there are times when she does feel unwell all over (a typical characteristic of rheumatoid arthritis as opposed to osteoarthritis, and fed up.

When I have a flare-up every bone feels hot and I feel generally unwell. I feel as if my hands are on fire. It's not a pleasant experience at all but at least I now know what it is so I can get on and deal with it. I put a packet of frozen peas on my legs, for example, and that does make me feel better.

Sometimes, though, I know I'm seventy-one, but having rheumatoid arthritis makes me feel like a very sad, and old, lady. I do get depressed – having a little cry now and then helps me when I feel sorry for myself. At least I do accept that this is me. And you know, I'm not as bad as some poor souls.

Like Isobel, twenty-six-year-old Gary, a trainee surveyor, believes he is one of the lucky ones – despite having had rheumatoid arthritis for the past fifteen years or so. It's likely that Gary first developed the disease when he was just seven years old. Severe cramp-like pains in his hip were initially put down to growing pains.

Most of my joints are affected now – my toes, ankles, knees, hands, elbows and shoulders. My back and hips are OK. The only obvious signs of deformity are a slight limp and I'm almost flat-footed. But at least I can get around and so I count myself lucky.

I wasn't diagnosed as having rheumatoid arthritis until I was eleven years old. By then I was showing signs of deformity. When I clenched my right hand, the knuckles of my middle fingers were much nearer my wrist than the others.

When I was told I had arthritis I wasn't devastated at all. Even at that age I was glad that my pains were given a definite cause and glad that at last I was going to be given medication that would stop the pain. And I was told that if I was a good boy and did my exercises everything would be fine.

As a means of safeguarding his joints, Gary was advised not to play contact sport, such as rugby or football, and told that he should swim or cycle.

> Had I been a rugby or football player anyway perhaps I would have minded. But I wasn't and I was lucky that my school had its own swimming pool. When the rest of the class had gym or games I went swimming. So I never felt left out and nobody ever teased me.
>
> I do play five-a-side football now at work. My ankles get very stiff and painful afterwards but I'm prepared to put up with that so that I can take part occasionally.

Coming to terms with arthritis hasn't really posed for Gary the great many problems it can for some sufferers.

> I've accepted I have the disease and that it's part of me. Having it from childhood means that I don't know any different kind of life. When I've spoken to older people who have been recently diagnosed they can be bitter because they can't do the things that they might have done before – whereas I probably haven't done them in the first place. I've always shied away from anything that would be too painful.
>
> I do try to do things though – like play five-a-side football. I'll always try to open a jam-jar first rather than immediately ask my wife to do it for me. I think if you give in to the disease you feel even worse. Of course, it depends on the person and the severity of the disease, but you definitely shouldn't wrap yourself up in cotton wool.

For Gary the most difficult thing to cope with is the pain.

It can take different forms. It can be a dull ache, a bit

like toothache that's always in the background. Or it can be a sudden stabbing pain. For me it's worse at night. That's when I notice it the most because my mind isn't occupied. Sleeping can be difficult, especially when I can't find a comfortable position.

I try to ignore it and you do get used to it. I imagine that if you gave my pain to a normally healthy person they'd take to their bed with it!

ANKYLOSING SPONDYLITIS

Ankylosing spondylitis (AS), also known as poker back or bamboo spine, is a rheumatic disease affecting the spine. It's one of a group of diseases referred to as seronegative spondarthropathies, which includes Reiter's syndrome (under the general umbrella of reactive arthritis); psoriatic arthritis and colitic arthritis. It affects just over one in a hundred people and is an inflammatory type of arthritis: 'ankylosing' means stiffening, 'spondylitis' means inflammation of the spine. It starts off insidiously over a period of weeks, usually at around the age of twenty to twenty-five. The pain stems from the sacroiliac joints which join the base of the spine to the pelvis. It is accompanied by stiffness and is normally felt in the lower back or perhaps as an ache in the buttocks. The pain and stiffness could be described as creeping and the bouts come and go, very often moving slowly further up the spine. It tends to be worse in the early morning. Joints of the back and hips are the main ones involved, but in a few cases shoulders, knees and ankles can be affected. Some sufferers experience a chest pain which is more severe when they breathe deeply. This pain stems from the joints between the ribs and the vertebrae.

Inflammation begins at the edges of the joints between the vertebrae. When the inflammation dies down, bone grows from both sides of the joint as part of a healing process. But eventually the bone can surround the joint completely, making it rigid. You may think there's a similarity here to rheumatoid arthritis because of the inflammation involved, but in ankylosing spondylitis the main inflammation is at the edge of the joints, where tendons and ligaments are attached to the bone, and also the inflammatory reaction causes scar tissue which eventually turns to bone.

The cause of ankylosing spondylitis, like so many forms of arthritis, is not known. It can run in families and is about three hundred times more common in people who have a certain genetic composition in the lymphocytes, the white blood cells that produce antibodies. The composition of genes is known as a marker and this one is named HLA B27. Without it you're unlikely to develop the disease. Only about one in ten of the population inherit this marker, and only two out of ten people with it will get ankylosing spondylitis.

It's well known that the disease often lessens in severity when people reach their fifties.

Interestingly, ankylosing spondylitis is considered to be one of the few rheumatic diseases that is more common in men and is nearly always thought of as a young man's disease. But experts now believe that, through misdiagnosis, ankylosing spondylitis is often missed in women. This misdiagnosis occurs because there is no simple blood test to confirm the disease's presence – as in the case of lupus (see page 40) – and x-rays don't always show up the damage for several years. The National Ankylosing Spondylitis Society (NASS) claims GPs often don't recognise the condition quickly enough and that it's not uncommon for there to be a period of eight years before its presence is diagnosed correctly.

Celia, a forty-five-year-old former teacher, knows only too well the pain and emotional turmoil caused by misdiagnosis. Her problem went undiagnosed for four years, despite her being in constant agony.

I was twenty-two when the first symptom started to appear. I thought I had strained a muscle in my right hip which wouldn't heal. The pain was so bad it made me scream in agony.

Celia was told she had a slipped disc by various hospital doctors. For four years she suffered. Not knowing what was wrong was almost as bad as putting up with the pain. Her work as a PE teacher was affected – in fact, she couldn't teach the subject any more and was lucky to work with sympathetic and supportive colleagues. At school they re-arranged classrooms so she could take her classes downstairs and Celia taught other subjects.

I lived around the condition. People accommodated the fact that there was indeed something very wrong with me. People carried me downstairs from my flat and got me to work.

As I used to teach PE I had some idea of how bodies worked and I knew there was something pretty grossly wrong with me. During that time I spent a lot of money searching for help. When you're not convinced of what you are being told and you haven't named the beast you search to try to explain it. I tried homoeopathy, reflexology, and osteopathy. I wanted to find out what was wrong with me so I could try to do something about it. I wasn't happy with the diagnosis of a slipped disc.

Finally it was contact with a chiropractor (see page 98) which triggered the correct diagnosis of her problem. The chiropractor refused to treat her and insisted she go to hospital for an x-ray to pinpoint exactly what was wrong. The x-ray showed she had ankylosing spondylitis. At the same time she had a blood test which showed she had the white blood cell marker HLA B27. Celia doesn't know anyone in her family who has had the disease.

Once diagnosed Celia took drugs targeting the disease. For the past sixteen or so years she has taken indomethacin and for the last three years she has experienced some long-term side-effects – anaemia, for example. 'Yet I'd totally seize up if I stopped the drugs so I have to carry on taking them,' she says.

Celia is also keen to stress that there are eye complications with ankylosing spondylitis. If you suffer from the disease you should discuss the possibility of suddenly developing an inflammation of the eye, called either iritis or anterior uveitis. It needs immediate treatment to prevent any permanent damage. Seek medical help immediately if you experience blurred vision, especially with pain, or if your eye is red around the coloured part (the iris) or even just generally red. It is thought that approximately four out of ten sufferers have experienced uveitis at some time, and some experts believe that sufferers should have eye-drops on hand in their refrigerators at all times in case of an attack.

Celia has had eye problems for the last four years and, because she hadn't been warned that eye inflammations were a complication of ankylosing spondylitis, she was in danger of losing her sight in one eye.

> It was very frightening. The pain was so bad I wanted to do anything to get rid of it. No one had told me about the eye trouble. At least I won't have to go through that experience again because I know the early warning signs. But not being able to see properly is still frightening. Sometimes it's as if I am looking through lots of net curtains at a window and I feel as if I want to move them away. At other times I just have extremely painful pressure building up.

As Celia points out, it's important to get medical treatment early on if you have ankylosing spondylitis. One of the primary objectives is to avoid the sufferer's spine becoming set in a bent position – the worst effect of the disease. As well as an x-ray, you may be tested for anaemia.

Also a test called the sedimentation rate may be carried out to establish how active the disease is.

The amount of damage done obviously depends on the severity of your symptoms. No two cases of the disease are the same. Some people have such mild symptoms they aren't even aware they have it.

The main treatment is exercise and anti-inflammatory drugs to help get rid of pain and stiffness. In severe cases surgery has been recommended to straighten the spine – although this is now rare. Radiotherapy is also rarely used as a means of pain control, but hip replacement surgery can be beneficial if the hip joints are badly damaged.

According to NASS you should learn their motto like a catechism: It's the doctor's job to relieve the pain and the patient's job to keep exercising and maintain a good posture. Celia has found that no matter how much it hurts at the time, exercise is really beneficial. You need to keep mobile to stop joints sticking. Ankylosing spondylitis differs from other forms of arthritis because the symptoms seem to be worse when a sufferer is resting.

> You have to learn to read your body and do exercises to strengthen muscles. You have to maximise the mobility you could possibly have. You end up having to be masochistic. If you don't move you get more seized up. You move when your body doesn't want to move. You have to inflict pain upon yourself to move parts of you that don't want to be moved at all, but two days later you'll be in a better condition than if you hadn't done it. You have to be tough to do that.

Patronising advice – from people who don't know what constant pain is or who haven't experienced the kind of disability that arthritis can cause – suggesting that ankylosing spondylitis shouldn't bring about too many problems and that most sufferers lead normal lives makes Celia angry. Her advice to other sufferers and those recently diagnosed is:

> Find out as much as you can and be prepared for a big shock. There's a lot of ignorance about it. NASS is helping in finding other sufferers. It can be very reassuring to talk to others in similar situations. Ankylosing spondylitis is insidious. It strikes young people when they have expectations of building up their life. It's pretty shattering to adjust your expectations and cope with the peer-group pressure.
>
> You should build up a dossier of information but learn to be discerning. In my opinion, there is a lot of rubbish written about ankylosing spondylitis – that it needn't interfere with your life or sexual relationships, for instance.
>
> I've found there are certain taboo areas, particularly the effects on relationships and particularly sexual relationships. I've talked to lots of other women with the disease who agree – if you've got hip trouble you can't have someone lying on top of you and it's also a strain on your partner anyway to see you in great pain. Arthritis does affect your life – every aspect of it.

People with arthritis have different ways of reacting emotionally to the disease. They can refuse to accept the diagnosis, and can be overwhelmed with despair or anger. Celia describes having arthritis as an experience similar to bereavement – the loss of part of your world is like losing a friend.

> You go through a grieving process – a sense of loss. Or I can be steaming angry at times. Sometimes I've felt that I couldn't care if I died in the night, that way it would be over. I've had depression about it – not

clinical depression. But I've felt so low, then I sleep, feel better and do lots of things.

I can drive and have a car and that keeps me sane. There are some days when I can't go out because my hips go a bit funny but I know it's only temporary. I've learned to live each day as it comes, then each morning as it comes, then each afternoon and evening.

PSORIASIS AND ARTHRITIS

I often receive letters asking me whether it's true that psoriasis and arthritis can sometimes be linked.

Psoriasis is a common and painful skin condition affecting more than a million people in the United Kingdom and the Republic of Ireland. It generally manifests itself in oval-shaped pieces of red skin covered with silvery scales on the elbows, knees, back and hands. It can become very painful on any part of the body liable to chafing. Most usually, psoriasis develops between the ages of fourteen and forty-five, very often during adolescence, pregnancy and the menopause. Having said that, it can disappear during these stages. It is neither contagious nor a result of poor standards of hygiene.

And *yes*, sufferers can develop arthritis. Psoriatic arthritis affects about 6 per cent of psoriasis sufferers. There's no link, however, between the location of the skin lesions and the location of the arthritic joints. In other words, the arthritis doesn't necessarily develop where the psoriasis is in evidence.

Psoriatic arthritis can be a crippling condition which restricts movement, most commonly in the hands, elbows and back, as well as causing inflammation, pain and tenderness in any joint. Joints near the fingertips can often be affected, with the fingernails taking on a pitted look. It is a similar condition to rheumatoid arthritis although generally milder: other symptoms include morning stiffness and fatigue.

Yet again, the cause is not known. Sometimes it will disappear for no apparent reason, while in other cases it will linger on. There is just no way of telling, unfortunately.

Many of you will, I'm sure, recall the most extreme form of this skin condition in the popular television drama *The Singing Detective*. The leading character had exfoliative dermatitis, which can also be a serious complication of other acute skin conditions. He also had psoriatic arthritis and was bedridden.

Barbara, a thirty-nine-year-old mother with three children, developed psoriasis as a teenager when her scalp became extremely dry and it seemed that she had a bad case of teenage dandruff. Soon after, she was told that she had psoriasis, an irritating skin condition, which would probably trouble her intermittently throughout her life.

The disease began to develop in red sore patches of skin on her elbows, knees and parts of her back. But it was when she became pregnant for the second time that psoriatic arthritis hit her with a vengeance right out of the blue.

Psoriasis sufferers can develop arthritis just as any other person can, although as I've said there is a very slight risk they could develop that particular type of arthritis known as psoriatic arthritis. Generally, psoriatic arthritis is a mild invasion of the joints, which can come and go, and even disappear. Sadly, Barbara has found that her arthritis has shown no signs of disappearing – although she still manages to fight both psoriasis and arthritis with spirit, courage and honesty.

> When my second daughter was born, it was as if the birth triggered something in my body, making normal movements impossible. Any move I made was agonising. My hands wouldn't move the way I wanted them to and my back was so stiff my husband had to push me out of bed in the mornings.

As many people with psoriasis know, there are considerable variations in how badly you can develop the condition. At best it can appear as several red patches of sore, scaly skin. At worst, it can become so widespread, a sufferer has to spend periods in hospital. But as far as Barbara is concerned psoriasis can be easier to live with than arthritis.

> When I first developed psoriatic arthritis, I have to say life with a toddler and a baby could have been better. Arthritis made me feel really useless. My fingers blew up like balloons. I couldn't pick up the baby or fasten nappy pins. I couldn't bend so I had to change her on top of the dining table. The joy of having her went because picking her out of the pram hurt me so much.
>
> I believe that arthritis is worse than psoriasis. It's now present throughout my body's joints particularly my right knee and right hip. They ache constantly.

As if Barbara hasn't had enough to cope with, she is also one of the tiny minority of people who have had hip replacement surgery which hasn't been as successful as she had hoped or desired. Following the replacement of her left hip her left leg is now longer than her right.

> That really set me back, It was such a shock. Even though the pain was relieved the day after the operation, my hopes crumbled. I'd never been warned that it might go wrong and that this might happen.
>
> Before the operation I was asked whether I wanted to be able bodied now and disabled in later life. And that because of my age, I'd probably need a second or even third replacement. In other words, live with the pain for a few years. But I couldn't. I was already at screaming point. I could hardly walk

but even then I was determined to keep on my feet.
I had things I wanted to do.

Now when I lie down at night my other hip hurts
and I'll probably need another replacement – but
then they might get it right next time.

Despite such severe setbacks Barbara has come to terms
with her arthritis to the extent that she tries to lead as
normal a family life as she can and refuses to give up or give
in to her problems.

What you've got, you've got to live with. It's no
good saying, 'if only'. You have to make the best of
what you have. Sometimes you get depressed but
that only makes the pain worse.

It has been found that about half of the people suffering
with psoriasis find that their skin problem becomes worse if
they're worried or under relentless pressure. For many this
can present a problem in the guise of a vicious circle. When
their psoriasis deteriorates this can make them worry even
more. Barbara has the added burden of discovering that
when her psoriasis worsens so does her arthritis.

If I get depressed about my arthritis, my psoriasis
gets worse. I've found that you need to talk to
someone or have someone to shout at – preferably
a friend. When times get bad, I tell a friend I've had
enough. You need to off-load your problem onto
someone else.

Talking to other sufferers has helped Barbara
enormously. For perhaps some ten years she'd suffered
without ever meeting another person with psoriasis. By
chance a newspaper headline changed her life. It read, 'The
P is silent and so are the sufferers.' This headline led her to
go to a meeting of psoriasis sufferers in her area.
For many people, the peace of mind that comes from

knowing they are not alone is essential to beat this condition because stress is recognised as a major factor in triggering and worsening psoriasis, which is one of the most common skin complaints.

> But the trouble with psoriasis and arthritis is that you're young and you want mentally to do more than you physically can which makes you cross and angry at yourself. Arthritis puts a strain on your marriage and your sex life. And I believe that needs saying more often – especially to the medical profession.
>
> When I had my hip replaced I had to ask what position would be safe for sex. Nobody offered practical help by speaking to me about it. People looked at me almost wondering why I was asking this question. But I was only in my thirties and I did have the rest of my life to live. In the end I was just given a note which mentioned four or five positions I'd never even heard of. I can honestly say that if I knew I'd become an arthritic I'd never have got married in the first place.

For many psoriasis sufferers the news that they have also developed arthritis can be very hard to accept. They may have only just come to terms with the skin disease.

COLITIS, CROHN'S DISEASE AND ARTHRITIS

Ulcerative colitis, a chronic inflammation of the colon, affects the large bowel; Crohn's disease largely affects, or inflames, the small intestine. They used to be seen as two separate conditions, but they are both inflammatory diseases of the alimentary canal – the long continuous hollow tube which stretches from the mouth right down to the anus – and neither is infectious. It's not an exaggeration to say that inflammatory bowel disease can affect any part of the digestive system because sometimes, though rarely, it is found in both the upper and lower sections of the alimentary canal, especially in Crohn's disease.

If the disease is extensive or severe, the sufferers may need to go to the loo as many as twenty times a day. Yet some may not experience much more than a little diarrhoea, perhaps stained with blood or mucus, and some occasional abdominal pain. Others may not realise anything is wrong until they need an emergency operation for acute abdominal pain, where the inflammation has blocked the passage of food. The disease is unpredictable and will usually follow a course of waxing and waning.

Nowadays, much more is being done, both medically and socially, to help sufferers. Thanks to the pioneering work of the National Association for Colitis and Crohn's disease (NACC), many sufferers now know that the disease can be managed and that it's nothing to be ashamed of. They also now know that theirs is not an uncommon condition. About one person in every thousand is a sufferer and the illness usually starts between the ages of sixteen and twenty-five.

The cause, however, is still not known. It could be that sufferers have an abnormal immune response in the colon, or that some kind of infection is the culprit. Contrary to popular opinion, the disease is not *caused* by stress or emotional upset – emotional upsets are usually a *result* of the disease. That's not to say that worry or a flu-type infection does not trigger an attack – this is highly likely. Just as, for instance, it's thought that bowel infections, colds and even taking antibiotics or perhaps pain-killing drugs, could set off an attack.

While the more common types of arthritis, osteoarthritis and rheumatoid are no more widespread in people with inflammatory bowel disease than anyone else, there are two types of arthritis which patients with Crohn's disease or ulcerative colitis do have a higher chance of developing.

As many as two out of ten sufferers have enteropathic arthritis, that is, due to bowel disease. This usually affects a large joint such as the knee, and pain and stiffness seem to be worse during a flare-up of the bowel disease. The attacks can come and go. This form of arthritis doesn't get worse and doesn't usually cause any deformities.

The second type of arthritis that colitis and Crohn's disease sufferers are at risk of developing is ankylosing spondylitis. (For more information, see page 18.) But unlike enteropathic arthritis, ankylosing spondylitis may begin years before the inflammatory bowel disease becomes apparent and the possible gradual worsening of symptoms doesn't have anything to do with how active the bowel disorder is.

The causes of these forms of arthritis aren't known, although it's thought that bacteria or certain parts of food absorbed from the inflamed bowel could be partly to blame.

Judith, a thirty-four-year-old sales representative, developed Crohn's disease when she was nineteen. Arthritis crept up on her about six years later.

> Friends and family were so surprised when they heard I had arthritis. Everyone said, 'At your age?' You automatically think arthritis is an old person's complaint.

So typical of arthritis and Crohn's disease, Judith found that her joint stiffness was much worse when her Crohn's disease was also niggling her.

> It definitely seemed to flare up when my Crohn's was bad. It was really nasty. We all get stiff but the stiffness of arthritis is something else. You have to experience it to really appreciate it.
>
> Sometimes I couldn't walk downstairs. I felt as if my shoes were filled with pebbles, no matter which shoes I wore. I had to hold on to the stair rail and come down one step at a time. This is bad enough in itself but when you have Crohn's disease you have to get to the loo fairly quickly.

First thing in the morning was the worst. My joints would be aching so much I felt as if I were a woman in her seventies. Just feeling old before your time is enough to make you depressed. All of my joints were affected – apart from my spine – and I thought I'd be suffering that way for the rest of my life which made me even more miserable.

Being positive about how she was going to cope encouraged Judith to carry on as normally as possible. Of course, she had to make quite a few changes in her life, from basics such as having a toilet installed in the upstairs of her home, to being forced to modify her car.

I had to change my car to an automatic one. When my arthritis was bad I couldn't change gears. To get the car into reverse I had to use both hands. I couldn't wind down the windows, so I had to have electric windows put at the front.

These fairly straightforward but expensive modifications did help to lessen the difficulties posed by her illness. Yet there were some things Judith was determined not to change.

I wasn't going to let arthritis dominate every aspect of my life. I liked country dancing and even though my knees were stiff and painful I thought positively. I was going to carry on doing the things I liked. Of course I couldn't do a lot of dancing in one go without sitting and resting in between but I wasn't going to stop either. I did feel that the exercise did me good.

Judith believes she coped by getting on with what she had to do. Through keeping busy she was able to forget the pain, once it had been damped down by her medication. Some people tell me that they dislike sharing experiences with others in similar situations, they prefer instead not to talk about their illness but try to ignore it. Judith was the opposite – she found talking to other sufferers most helpful.

> Knowing you're not the only one is so important. I knew, too, that there were other people much worse off than me – so who was I to complain?

But arthritis did affect her feelings about being a wife.

> I suppose you could describe the way I felt at the time as inadequate. I saw other women working and doing the housework and I felt terrible because I couldn't do that. My husband, Gerry, was at work all day, then when he came home he'd have to help out.
>
> I couldn't do the cooking very often or the ironing, or take the ironing basket upstairs. I couldn't bear any weight on my wrists. Gerry had to come to the supermarket with me. I couldn't lift any shopping or walk very far without my knees or ankles giving way. There were some things I loved and couldn't do any more.
>
> I love making a Christmas fruit cake but in the end I even had to get Gerry to help me do that. Obviously he has stronger wrists and could stir the mixture, because for me it was impossible. Things began happening to me that you'd associate with an elderly person not a woman in her twenties.

For Gerry, a forty-three-year-old salesman, seeing his young wife in pain and discomfort was frustrating.

> You can't do anything really for a person in such pain, other than help with things like shopping or whatever else she wants. And I have to be honest and say that at times I do feel helpless. It was a shock, too, initially to discover that someone so

young should have such restriction of movement in
their joints.

Judith was, to some extent, fortunate that the anti-
inflammatory drug, indomethacin, did control her arthritis.

> Without drugs I would have been in excruciating
> pain. For me the pain of arthritis was worse than
> that of Crohn's. It's a pain I don't ever want again
> and certainly wouldn't wish on anyone.
>   With Crohn's, I had a burning sensation down
> the right-hand side of my abdomen – as if someone
> had stuck a red-hot poker into me and left it there.
> With arthritis, every time I moved a joint I'd feel a
> sharper pain.

Relief from arthritis came for Judith four years ago
following surgery for Crohn's disease. Many sufferers find
that treating the inflammatory bowel disease in this way
does relieve their joint pain. It's possible that a local cause or
by-product of the bowel inflammation provokes the
arthritis.

For Judith it was an extremely welcome relief and it all
happened pretty quickly.

> In a matter of a few weeks I noticed a tremendous
> improvement. Once I'd recuperated from the oper-
> ation I found I could gradually do a lot more. I didn't
> need drugs and I began to feel my 'young' old self
> again. It was great and has been ever since – touch
> wood.

GOUT

Gout, or acute gouty arthritis, is a common and an
extremely painful form of arthritis, described to me as a
'tormenting pain'. The difference between gout and other

forms of arthritis is that gout is treated as something of a joke by those who know nothing about it and who have never experienced it. A sad fact of life that does nothing to cheer up an agonised gout sufferer.

Unlike many other forms of arthritis, the cause is known. Gout is an inflammatory reaction caused by uric acid crystals deposited in the joints, which trigger a reaction in the tissue. It begins as a sensation of discomfort, rapidly developing into excruciating pain. The joint then becomes acutely inflamed and can turn bluish-red and shiny. It is almost too tender to be touched. Gout can lead to joint damage if deposits stay and build up in the joints over a number of years.

Gouty people have a faulty system for breaking down and excreting the waste products from protein food particles (purines). Normally these waste products, particularly broken-down uric acid – is passed out in our urine but in an attack of gout uric acid builds up in the blood. Most of us pass out enough of these wastes to reduce the amount in our blood and keep the levels low. People with gout have a tendency to higher levels of uric acid than normal – either they don't pass out enough, perhaps because of drugs or damage to the kidney, or they produce too much. Sometimes the high levels can be caused by eating or drinking too much, so over-producing uric acid in the body.

When there is too much uric acid in the blood, it can adhere in crystal form to the usually smooth membranes that lubricate the joints' surfaces, making them like sandpaper. The crystals can also drop into the joint space to cause inflammation, swelling and pain – that's when it appears swollen, hot and red. Any movement of the joint is extremely painful.

The attack normally lasts for a few days while the cells in the lining try to get rid of the crystals. The joint then gradually goes back to normal. The usual pattern is that the attack starts off at night for no obvious reason. Occasionally a sufferer is aware that an infection such as a common cold, or even knocking your toe, can trigger an attack. So can taking diuretics.

Deposits of crystals, called tophi, can be seen under the skin around the ears in frequent sufferers. In severe cases, there may be some joint deformity and loss of movement and crystals may also collect in the kidneys. Consequently, the aim of treatment is to prevent joint destruction, tophic formation and renal damage.

Not everyone with higher levels of uric acid develops gout: some people may have just one or two attacks in their life while others experience repeated bouts involving joint after joint. Gout often runs in families. It's sometimes said that sufferers are very intelligent although I'm not sure how necessarily true this is!

It's seven times more common in men than women, probably because levels of uric acid are generally higher in men. More than seven out of ten cases involve the big toe – goodness knows why. Most often, no other joints are affected at the same time, though the feet, ankles, knees, wrists or fingers can be affected.

Gout can be detected fairly easily by a blood test. Occasionally a sample of the fluid in the affected joint will be tested for uric acid crystals to confirm the diagnosis, although most doctors can spot classic symptoms of gout at a glance, as in the case of John, a sixty-two-year-old, semi-retired sales engineer.

The typical age for the onset of gout is during the thirties and forties. John was forty-six when he had his first attack.

It came on really suddenly right out of the blue and I'd certainly never experienced anything like it before.

I woke up one morning with such pain and stiffness in the big toe of my left foot. I couldn't believe how big it was when I looked at it. It was honestly twice as big as its normal size. The skin was cherry red, tender and shiny – as well as *feeling* as if it was going to explode, it *looked* as if it was going to explode.

What's more, I couldn't move my foot at all. I couldn't bear any pressure on it. It was absolutely agonising. I had no idea then what was wrong.

I'd been to my brother's wedding the day before and I thought that perhaps I'd knocked my toe while I was dancing. I had to drive home a few days later, from Cheltenham to Sheffield, in excruciating pain and trying to use only my right foot! And to try to get to bed I had to crawl on my hands and knees at the same time as holding my foot away from the floor.

After a week of torture I finally saw my doctor. He immediately diagnosed gout. What surprised me at the time was the way gout, a form of arthritis, provoked laughter and constant teasing. Friends thought it was very funny and teased me that it was a rich man's complaint and that I obviously had another life as a country squire eating lots of game and supping plenty of port.

Neither my wife nor my daughter were sympathetic. They thought I'd brought it on myself and that it was my own fault so I ought to keep quiet about it. They didn't understand that the way my body dealt with uric acid wasn't my fault at all.

John took his doctor's advice to cut down on fat although he found dieting very difficult. Six months later he had another supposedly unprompted attack in exactly the same manner as before – except this time the big toe on his right foot was affected.

I couldn't sleep because of the pain. I had to rest my foot on a pillow it throbbed so much. I couldn't bear any blankets to touch it so I had to try to sleep with my foot out of bed.

There was no way I could have got to work. I'd

just keep still and hope the pain would go away. Any movement which disturbed the joint resulted in terrible pain.

John had four more attacks at intervals of six to nine months, which was when he began to take allopurinol regularly (a drug which reduces the level of uric acid in the blood). He's taken it successfully ever since.

At that time I used to get little swellings behind my ears. They weren't painful just irritating. It was the pain of a gout attack that I just couldn't cope with. It would mean I was out of action for a week at least. My finger joints and knees began to be affected as well, although the pain in my fingers wasn't as bad as in my feet. But my knee was terrible. It would be red and swollen which meant I couldn't walk at all.

Looking back I did also eat the wrong things. I'd eat liver and bacon about twice a week I enjoyed it so much, and I'd drink lots of wine. I now know that liver has a high purine content so I hardly ever eat it and I drink alcohol in moderation as well as making sure I take in plenty of water. I don't worry about having to take tablets because I'd do anything rather than suffer that pain again.

As I've already pointed out, most gout sufferers are men, and it's usually only after the menopause that women are prone to the condition. But the idea that only overweight, alcohol-addicted Colonel Blimps are affected is a fallacy. Even children can develop the disease, so badly they can suffer kidney failure. Young sufferers have an enzyme defect which leads to an over-production of uric acid. This can be deposited in the joints and can also damage kidneys. Research is currently underway to find a defective gene believed to be responsible for the condition.

The outlook for the gout sufferer is good. Untreated, an attack can last days or even weeks but will eventually subside. Some people will be lucky and just have a single attack, others will have another after a long interval. More often, though, attacks increase in frequency and may even merge into each other. As attacks heighten, the affected joints can become damaged and this in turn adds to the pain.

As we can clearly see from John's account, the condition can be controlled by drugs (see section on treatment, page 49), resting the affected joint and raising it slightly, as well as watching your diet and losing weight. Perhaps surprisingly, a heavy meal is as likely to trigger an attack as over-indulgence in alcohol.

Should you experience severe pain in your big toe, don't automatically assume that you must have knocked it. But don't automatically think it's gout either. Let your doctor decide what the problem is. You'll probably need treatment of some sort, whatever the cause, and a correct diagnosis is essential – first, to rule out septic arthritis (caused by a germ getting into the joint leading to inflammation), which would need antibiotics, or injury, or even rheumatoid arthritis, and second, to prevent long-term damage of joints, which would result in lots more pain as well as possible kidney stones or kidney damage.

So never ignore a painful joint, no matter how much dancing you've done at a wedding the night before.

SYSTEMIC LUPUS ERYTHEMATOSUS (SLE)

This is one of a group of diseases called 'collagen' or connective tissue diseases. It's an auto-immune disease like rheumatoid arthritis, but in this case the body's defences abnormally attack its own tissues not just in the joints but also widely in the body. They attack its connective tissues – those tissues, like fibres for example, that are responsible for holding all the other tissues together and in place. As yet we don't really know why the attack occurs.

Collagen diseases are rare and include systemic sclerosis – scleroderma – when the skin is mainly affected; polymyositis and dermatomyositis (rare diseases causing a skin and muscle inflammation); and polyarteritis nodosa (PAN), a very rare disease which causes patches of inflammation in the walls of small- and medium-sized arteries.

Most people have probably never even heard of the rheumatic disorder lupus, even though it's more common than multiple sclerosis. It is a chronic inflammatory disease that most commonly affects the joints – causing the arthritis – but also the skin, heart, kidneys and central nervous system, indeed, any of the body's soft tissues, may be involved. The inflammation arises, as I've said, when the body's natural defence system, its antibody system, attacks its own connective tissues. The antibodies (blood proteins) designed to protect the body, say from bacteria, attack the sufferer instead.

Arthritis is only one aspect of the disease's symptoms (although it's estimated that more than 95 per cent of people with lupus have joint problems). Others include extreme fatigue, described by sufferers as the type of tiredness that wouldn't be helped even if you could sleep twenty-four hours a day; muscle aches; anaemia; oral ulcers; a general sense of being unwell and chest pains because of the inflammation of the lining of the lungs. It can also destroy important organs, sometimes the kidneys.

When lupus is 'active', sufferers say it's as if they are going through a bad bout of flu because their joints and muscles ache so much. Most lupus sufferers experience these aches and pains because, like rheumatoid arthritis, the joints become inflamed. Yet the inflammation in lupus rarely causes damage to the joints, as is the case in rheumatoid arthritis.

More women than men suffer from lupus – in fact, as many as nine women to one man. It's thought that one in two thousand women suffer from lupus, usually in their child-bearing years from fifteen to fifty. Just as there's an exception to every rule, however, so there is with lupus, for children and even newborn babies can be affected.

Women with lupus have an increased chance of

miscarriage. If you suffer from lupus and are thinking of becoming pregnant get your doctor's advice. Your drug treatment will need careful monitoring or may even be modified. The disease may become active again during pregnancy and just after the birth.

Like ankylosing spondylitis, lupus can often go undiagnosed. The charity Lupus UK claims some people have suffered for twenty years without being diagnosed correctly and much more information and awareness of the problem is needed. Part of the difficulty in diagnosing lupus in the past has been because it varies so much from patient to patient and because of the disease's ability to mimic other diseases. It is, in fact, sometimes known as the 'great impersonator'. Patients have been told they were suffering from growing pains, glandular fever, even severe migraine. Symptoms can also wax and wane, and sometimes disappear altogether. Yet there is a simple blood test, called the anti-nuclear factor antibody test, that can be carried out to establish the presence of the disease.

The cause is unknown. The fact that women are affected nine times more often than men, that lupus is common among women of childbearing age and that it's unusual for it to develop before a woman's menstrual periods begin strongly suggests that female hormones play a prominent part in the illness. And experts now believe that there's a genetic predisposition which can be sparked off by triggers such as a viral infection or ultraviolet light. About one third of lupus sufferers are photosensitive (sensitive to sunlight) and develop skin rashes and lesions after exposure to the sun. The disease is common in sunny climates, but even in this country sufferers should be sure to use high-protection sun-block creams which protect against UVA and UVB rays and to wear protective clothing, especially a sun hat. Lupus sufferers have written to me about working in offices, and whether they should be careful when coming into contact with fluorescent lighting. The answer is yes, because that, too, emits some ultraviolet rays.

Lupus, or SLE, used to be considered a life-threatening

disease which progressively increased in severity. Today, for most patients, it can be controlled, usually with drugs such as steroids, anti-malarials and sometimes immuno-suppressive drugs. Aspirin is often taken for pain relief.

Although the understanding of lupus and other auto-immune conditions, like rheumatoid arthritis, does get better every year, the most successful treatment is still steroids. These powerful drugs can dampen down the worst, if not all, of the symptoms. What's more, modern research has shown that the earlier the condition is diagnosed the better the outcome will be. It's as if by dousing the activities of lupus early on, the full damage it could otherwise do is kept in check.

Rose, a fifty-year-old former staff nurse, has lupus and, in particular, extremely painful joints: 'I've had lupus for more than thirty years, starting off with aches and pains, funny abdominal pain, dreadful colds and fatigue,' she says.

Lupus was diagnosed some time after Rose had a stillborn baby and her Achilles' tendons seized up so severely she was unable to walk. 'Initially I was told I had rheumatoid arthritis, but my nurse's training told me I had something other than that.'

The disease has such a wide variety of symptoms that some sufferers don't have arthritis at all, or, if they do, the arthritis doesn't always cause joint damage. But Rose's joint pain became progressively worse as she found her arthritis flitted from joint to joint. Her knees, hips, shoulders and elbows have all been stiff and painful. Walking has been almost impossible at times and she's been forced to walk on tiptoe. Her hands have regularly been swollen. The tips of her fingers point downwards and her little fingers splay outwards. The thumb joint on her left hand has been dislocated.

> One elbow at a time would lock. It was painful but awkward more than anything else. It would lock in a wide v-shape, with my hand halfway up to my shoulders – for as long as a week before easing off.

The bones in her feet are misplaced – sometimes she has a trapped nerve in her foot.

> And that's when I go into orbit. Yet, I have more function in my hands and fingers than someone with rheumatoid arthritis would have at this stage. It's difficult to bend my fingers – but that's just a matter of adapting now. I try not to lift heavy things. I push rather than lift where possible. I fill a kettle using a jug rather than pick up the kettle and hold it under the tap.
>
> I have to admit I should make more use of aids – the types suggested by occupational therapists – around the home. I'm a bit stubborn and still want to do things myself and my own way. It's vanity I suppose, in addition to not wanting to give in to lupus.

Rose has had such bad flare-ups of the disease she's been in hospital on several occasions. Two years ago she had a particularly bad time. 'Every bit of me seemed to be affected,' she recalls. 'I felt as though I had gravel between my scalp and my skull. My lungs and heart were affected. And I had chronic renal failure.' After that Rose had an abdominal cyst which had to be removed, followed by removal of her gall bladder.

> Since then I've steadily improved. I don't have as much pain in my joints apart from when I get overtired. My feet are still sore all the time though.
>
> I'm a firm believer in taking vitamins. I also always use a sunscreen. Just because I live in the north of Scotland doesn't mean I can go without it.
>
> I do believe it's important for lupus sufferers to listen to their body. To rest when their body tells them to. I know it's difficult, especially if you have a young family, which because of the usual age lupus strikes is very likely.

When I was a young mother, when my little boy slept so did I. If you force yourself to go out shopping when you're tired you only end up more tired. I find when I'm overtired I can't sleep because my mind is still racing.

This sensation of an active mind and an exhausted body is described by many sufferers. Some say it's as though your mind has had an extra strong coffee and your body's had a sleeping tablet.

Even when you feel fine don't overdo things. If your house is untidy then it's untidy. If people come to see you then, remember, it's you they're coming to visit not your house. You'll only suffer more in the long term and you'll then take longer to feel well again if you do. You should pace yourself. And don't forget there's always tomorrow. You have to enjoy life within the disease's limits.

As well as conventional treatment, from aspirin to steroids, Rose has tried alternatives and has found spiritual healing of immense benefit no matter what sceptics might say. She's now a spiritual healer herself.

Healers are very caring people. Their aim after all is to help heal someone. People are so calm and relaxed after a healing. You sit in a chair with your feet firmly on the ground. You relax, shut your eyes and the healer holds his or her hands over the crown of your head. Some people feel sensations of heat, or cold, tingling, or pins and needles. I felt both heat and cold and even saw a bright light in front of my eyes – it was just like seeing the sun glowing. It was a beautiful sensation.

The healing process goes through the healer to you. Some people explain it as universal energy, some believe it's God.

Whatever the explanation – if it brings any relief it's to be welcomed. Make sure the healer is 'recognised' and so is not a charlatan, and that he or she charges a reasonable rate. Many healers won't accept a fee, perhaps believing that their powers are God-given.

Rose believes that her will to recover has also helped her to survive. From the outset she wasn't going to live the life of an invalid nor was she going to give up hope.

> I've always maintained that lupus wasn't going to get the better of me. I was going to keep active for as long as I could. I hope to have a good few years yet – I've got a lot of living to do.

ARTHRITIS AND TREATMENT

While it's true that there is no cure, it's false to think that nothing can be done to relieve the symptoms of arthritis. There is a great deal of research going on and I'll mention just a few examples to give you an idea of how much energy is being put into the quest for better treatment and a cure.

British scientists are working on perfecting longer-lasting artificial joints, for example. Trials in Israel on patients with arthritis of the knee found that low-power light emitters helped ease pain significantly when administered to both sides of the knee over ten days. Also scientists are hopeful that in the next twenty years or so they will develop a vaccine for people who they believe are susceptible to arthritis. The Arthritis and Rheumatism Council has given grants to back all manner of research projects into arthritis, from investigating the body's immune response in relation to rheumatoid arthritis to searching for infection triggers, both in ankylosing spondylitis and other types of arthritis.

Treating arthritis is still for many people a question of trial and error. It will probably take time to find the right treatment for you because some things work for some people. Don't worry unduly about taking drugs because they may produce side-effects – try them first. You mustn't fear that a specialist will necessarily want to give you steroids – they are usually only prescribed as a last resort. What matters is that you are relieved of pain and inflammation and that something is done to stop your arthritis worsening. And steroids do far, far more good than harm, although many people, understandably, worry about the side-effects. It's because they are such powerful medicines that, should large doses need to be given for long periods when nothing else will do, side-effects may be experienced. It's important to take the dose suggested – if you skimp on it it won't be able to do its good work and you won't get the blessed relief from pain and other symptoms.

Most people with arthritis are cared for by their GP and about a quarter are referred to a rheumatologist (a specialist in rheumatic diseases) or an orthopaedic surgeon (a specialist in the repair of joint damage). Being referred by your GP to a rheumatologist in a hospital carries with it the on-the-spot bonus of ready help from other key people, such as physiotherapists and occupational therapists and chiropodists.

WHEN TO SEEK HELP AND WHAT TO SAY

The symptoms of arthritis vary widely from type to type and even from person to person. Just because you have arthritis the effects aren't necessarily going to be severe. But if you experience persistent pain in one or more joints, don't ignore it and soldier on, go to your doctor as soon as you can so you can get an accurate diagnosis.

Major joints, such as the hips, knees and ankles, are naturally in constant use, so you can expect some slight aches and pains now and then. Yet it's important to see your GP if you are concerned, particularly if the pain doesn't seem to go away. Sometimes you may have arthritis in a hip joint but won't be aware of it because you feel pain in your knee, which is why joint pain should always be checked out by a doctor. If you do have arthritis the sooner treatment is started the better.,

I must stress again that the information contained in this book is not intended for self-diagnosis but as a guide to understanding the disease and how other sufferers cope. If you have not yet been diagnosed but suspect you may have some kind of arthritis, see your doctor. You may also need to see a specialist, and may need a number of tests to try to establish what sort of arthritis you have. For example, the ESR (Erythrocyte Sedimentation Rate) can yield information on the presence and degree of rheumatoid arthritis.

Your blood may also be tested for a substance called rheumatoid factor which is present in the blood of about eight out of ten rheumatoid arthritis sufferers. The rheumatoid factors – there are more than one – are anti-bodies circulating in the blood which are involved in the causation of the disease. X-rays may also be taken to find out how much damage has been done.

If you know you have arthritis you should still visit your doctor on a fairly regular basis so that any worsening of symptoms can be dealt with as soon as they occur.

I understand that it's hard to keep faith in the medical profession if nothing improves your condition, but remember doctors aren't mind-readers and you are the only person who can explain just how you are feeling, how much pain you are in and whether treatment – be it physiotherapy or drugs – is affecting you.

You may say that your doctor never listens to you but he could sometimes equally say you never talk to him. When describing your symptoms, first tell him the worst ones. Then give brief, clear details. If your treatment isn't working, say so.

No matter how rushed your doctor may seem, it's still important for you to make the most of the time you've got with him. So there's absolutely no harm in preparing yourself mentally for a visit. It helps many people to write down a list of questions, or a list of things they don't understand and would like explained in more detail or more simply. A tip though – try to keep your questions short and to the point. Don't waste time waffling on. Very often just knowing you have the list in your pocket or handbag will give you such confidence you won't even need to refer to it!

Talking of lists, I know one patient who has written down every drug and every form of treatment and operation she has had for the last eighteen years. She finds it invaluable as it's impossible to remember off-hand the names of some of the anti-inflammatory medicines she's been given and how she reacted to them. She's also noted the exact dates of the several surgical procedures she's undergone. Keeping a 'medical diary' could be a useful reference book for you, too.

I know it's an easy thing to say, but don't allow yourself to be intimidated by medical staff. If you don't understand what you're being told, make sure they realise this and ask for it to be explained more slowly, or more simply. You needn't feel embarrassed or stupid. You certainly won't be the first person they're seen who's had difficulty grasping all the facts. And you won't be the last, either.

If you're worried about something in particular, make sure you ask questions about it. Very often some reassurance is all you might need. There's nothing worse than anxiety that stems from ignorance.

It's not unknown for someone seeing a doctor to remember only about a third of what they've been told. One sufferer told me this regularly happened to her and her advice is to take a friend or partner along with you. That way you feel less intimidated and what you don't remember your friend often does.

Medication and you – if your doctor thinks you'll benefit from medication, then you ought to give it a chance by taking the drugs exactly as instructed. You can always double-check with your pharmacist if you can't remember everything your doctor told you. Your pharmacist can also explain more about the drug – how it works and the likelihood of any side-effects.

If you do experience side-effects – a rash, for example, or an upset stomach – contact your doctor immediately and ask his advice. It may be possible to switch to another drug. Don't suddenly stop taking it.

When you are prescribed a medication, always mention if you are already taking something else. The two may not mix and could be dangerous.

Give your medication a chance – don't expect immediate miracles. It may take a little time to find the one most effective for you, so be sure to tell your doctor if you don't feel any better after a while.

DRUGS

Drugs are used effectively to treat arthritis by greatly reducing pain and inflammation. But sometimes hitting on the right drug for you is a question of trial and error because, as I've said, what's acceptable to one person may not suit another.

There are many types of non-steroidal anti-inflammatory drugs available. They work by inhibiting the production of prostaglandins, which pass on pain signals to the brain. Examples of ones used in the treatment of arthritis are mild pain relievers like aspirin or ibuprofen (Nurofen), or drugs such as naproxen, mefenamic acid (Ponstan) and indomethacin. Indomethacin is one of the most popular and widely prescribed drugs in the treatment of arthritis as it seems to be effective time and again.

These non-steroidal anti-inflammatory drugs are quite commonly prescribed in order to reduce pain and inflammation. Aspirin can irritate the stomach and if used excessively can cause bleeding, so it shouldn't be taken if you have a stomach ulcer or other stomach disorder. Excess use can also cause tinnitus (constant noises or ringing sensations in the ear). Analgesics are also used for pain relief, although they don't help inflammation – examples are paracetamol and the opiate codeine. Paracetamol can be useful when a person is intolerant of aspirin.

Aspirin, however, isn't given for the treatment of gout because the level of uric acid in the body can be raised by it. Instead Colchicine, an old drug used since the eighteenth century and once extracted from the autumn crocus flower, is often prescribed for gout. Others are allopurinol (usually for long-term treatment to prevent recurrent attacks) which stops too much uric acid forming in the first place; and probenecid which helps the kidneys to increase the amount excreted and so aid the prevention of further attacks.

Anti-rheumatic drugs help stop or slow down the disease process although why they do so is not entirely understood.

They work more slowly than anti-inflammatory drugs and sometimes it takes quite a while before any benefit is noticed. Examples of these are gold-based drugs (such as sodium aurothiomalate and auranofin), penicillamine and more recently sulphasalazine, the anti-malarial drug chloroquine (used in the treatment of rheumatoid arthritis and lupus) and also immunosuppressives like methotrexate. Immunosuppressives work by suppressing cells thought to cause the damage in arthritis and are used only when absolutely necessary.

Steroids (corticosteroid drugs) can also be used effectively to reduce inflammation. They occur naturally in the body but can be man-made. They are the most powerful of all anti-inflammatory medicines and are used when the body tissue becomes so inflamed and swollen that it is very painful. They bring relief by reducing the swelling, which is stretching the tissues and causing pain, and by cooling the tissues, which is soothing.

Steroids also dampen the body's defence system – its anti-bodies – so they are especially useful in auto-immune diseases like rheumatoid arthritis where the body's defences attack its own tissues, in this case the joints.

Sometimes steroids are taken in tablet form but they can be administered by an injection into the joint. The injection is the best way of gaining the benefits of steroids without the whole body receiving a dose, therefore keeping side-effects to a minimum.

Drugs given in the treatment of arthritis are carefully monitored – sometimes by regular blood tests because of possible side-effects. For instance, anti-rheumatic drugs can cause rashes and digestive disturbances, or even kidney damage. Steroids can make you retain fluid, increase your appetite or cause mood swings.

SURGERY

Don't think of surgery as a last resort. It's a useful way of relieving severe arthritis.

There are many surgical procedures carried out to ease arthritis. Possible operations include a synovectomy to remove the lining of the affected joint – usually the knee – so the area of inflammation is taken away in a bid to prevent further joint damage. Also bone can be removed to ease pain, damaged tendons can be repaired and joints can be replaced. A joint replacement operation isn't carried out without first exploring other means of treatment, however.

The joints of the knees, ankles, shoulders, elbows, wrists and fingers can all be replaced. Surgeons can now perform replacement surgery on diseased knuckles, for instance, using artificial joints made from flexible silicone rubber which should last for the rest of the patient's life. This is particularly useful when a patient suffers from a condition known as ulnar drift, which causes knuckles to deteriorate and the tendons that normally run over the top of the joints to slip sideways and down, pulling the fingers to the right or left.

Thousands of people who might once have faced life in a wheelchair or who could have become bedridden have now been given new mobility thanks to modern techniques of joint replacement. A total hip replacement operation is the most common and successful of all replacement operations. Called an arthroplasty, it has given a new lease of life to a great many people since it was developed.

In the operation the old arthritic ball and socket joint is completely removed, the socket re-lined with tough plastic material cemented into place and a new, round, stainless steel head is fitted to the thigh bone. The round head has a tail which is slimmer than the top of your femur (thigh bone) and is placed into the middle of the bone. The head swivels in a plastic socket. The joints are made from specially formulated metal and plastics which aren't normally rejected by the body's immune system and which don't themselves react to the body's tissues.

The operation works successfully in old and young patients, but usually if someone in need of a hip replacement is younger than normal, surgeons will use different techniques – often necessitating a long hospital stay – to give the union of the new joint longer life.

More than 40,000 people in the UK have had a hip replaced. And interestingly, farmers seem to number high amongst them. According to a recent report in the *British Medical Journal*, farming doesn't seem to be the healthy occupation it is often perceived as. Research has now shown that farmers are eight times more likely than office workers to suffer osteoarthritis in the hip. That means that about one in five farmers needs a hip replacement!

Fortunately, the operation's success rate is excellent: there is a 95 per cent chance that it will get rid of pain totally. Following a successful replacement most people find to their delight that they eventually regain about three-quarters of a normal hip joint's mobility. Their dreams of pain-free movement and activities such as running, cycling and even tennis are usually possible once again.

You should be up and about within a few days of the operation and able to go home in two to three weeks. Getting over the operation and how quickly you become mobile again will depend on your mental attitude and your willingness to follow the advice of physiotherapists (see page 55). Their exercises are a major part of rehabilitation.

Recovery will also depend to some extent on your age and how fit you are. If you are at all overweight, use any time you have before the operation to shed those excess pounds, as this will make the all-important walking exercises afterwards considerably easier. I think you will be surprised and delighted at how soon you are able to resume a normal, active life.

When Bubbles was sixty-one she had a hip replacement operation which banished the pain of osteoarthritis in her hip once and for all. That was ten years ago and she was so thrilled by the surgery's transformation of her life that she still keeps her operation stitches as a memento.

Bubbles had suffered from osteoarthritis for about twenty years before, finally, the pain in her hip grew too much to bear and walking became impossible.

The pain was there constantly. I felt if I could get my hand inside my joint I would be able to rub the pain away. I could hardly walk before the operation, I even had to go upstairs on my bottom if I wanted to use the bathroom because I couldn't walk up steps.

When I was shown an x-ray of my hip it looked just like the surface of the moon. The bone seemed to be covered with dark craters. [What Bubbles saw were areas of irregularity which show up darker on an x-ray film.]

When a joint replacement was offered I was delighted. I would have accepted anything by then to take away that pain and to be able to walk again.

I wasn't frightened by the thought of surgery. When you get to my age you don't worry about dying, you worry about how you're going to die. So in the unlikely event of anything happening to me on the operating table I reckoned that way I wouldn't know anything about it.

In fact, Bubbles was amazed at the speed of her recovery and how effective the replacement was at relieving the pain.

I was in hospital for fourteen days in all and I can honestly say that when I came round from the operation I didn't feel any pain any more. The nurses offered me painkillers but I didn't need them. I was overjoyed – I couldn't believe my luck. I have osteoarthritis in my knee too but I didn't even notice that pain.

Three days later I was walking up the ward with

the help of two sticks and my hip has been fine ever since.

Knee joint replacements are also on the increase, and are very successful at relieving pain. Currently about half as many knee joints are replaced as hip joints. New knee joints called 'condylar joints' mean replacements are more efficient than they used to be. Knee replacements don't seem to work as well in younger people, though, as they tend to be more active and this puts too much strain on the new joint.

I regularly receive letters asking about the possibility of a shoulder joint replacement operation. Yes they are possible and in many, if not all, regions of the country there are orthopaedic surgeons who will undertake such a replacement when this is required. However, most conditions that affect the shoulder joint are not actually due to the joint itself, but to the muscles, tendons and soft tissues around it.

If it is decided to replace the joint, the pain should still disappear but the drawback is that the replacement joint is not as flexible. The healthy shoulder joint is the most mobile of all joints in the body because of its brilliant system of muscles and pulleys. The shallow saucer-like ball and socket hinge enables the shoulder to achieve its great swivelling ability – to understand what I mean, just move your arms around and notice the range of movement. Because a replacement isn't so manoeuvrable, there is considerable restriction of shoulder movement.

But the great advantage of this procedure is in pain relief – which is, of course, a highly desirable end in itself.

I must point out, however, that joint replacements do sometimes fail. They can become loose or infected, and when this happens the replacement joint usually has to be removed.

PHYSIOTHERAPY

Many arthritis sufferers find physiotherapy extremely helpful, soothing and relaxing. In this way, and others, physiotherapy plays a vital role in the treatment of arthritis and it could be that you come into more regular contact with your physiotherapist than your doctor or specialist. Many patients have told me that they prefer to discuss their problems with a physiotherapist, or occupational therapist, rather than with a doctor. I'm told they seem less intimidating and less in a rush!

Physiotherapy covers a wide range of techniques. The physiotherapist will usually work out an individual course of treatment for each patient. And, of course, he or she will need to chat to you about how much mobility you have and how bad your arthritis is. He or she will assess the state of your muscles and joints before embarking on your course of treatment as the whole point of physiotherapy is to relieve pain and to try to improve your muscle tone and the range of movements your joints are able to make.

Isobel, who suffers from severe rheumatoid arthritis, as we've mentioned on page 14, was very impressed when her physiotherapist spent three-quarters of an hour examining her joints and establishing exactly what her range of movements was. 'She wriggled my ankles to see what movement I had. Then she did the same with my knees and worked her way around my body.' Just by doing this, Isobel's physiotherapist made her feel much more at ease, and more confident that she wouldn't force her to make movements she wasn't capable of. Because of this she felt she could trust her that much more and not be frightened to follow her directions. 'I really want to urge people not to be frightened of physiotherapy,' Isobel says. 'Help yourself by being helped.'

There are many modalities of treatment used for the benefit of arthritis sufferers in addition to exercise programmes. Examples are ice; hot-packs; wax; interferential therapy (a method of using electric current to ease pain by interrupting the pain reception network as well as stimulating circulation to reduce inflammation); ultrasonic (a therapy using sound waves at high frequencies pointed at an affected area to help relax muscles, reduce inflammation, encourage healing and numb pain); infra-red (a form of deep-heat treatment); laser; traction (a means of stretching); Faradic footbaths; and transcutaneous nerve stimulators (or TENS machines) used by many specialists to relieve pain due to arthritis and back pain. Oxygen therapy is sometimes used for treating arthritic patients with leg ulcers.

A TENS machine is a small battery-powered unit which you strap around you, positioning the contact points over the painful area before switching it on. A low-frequency signal then stimulates the brain into producing its own natural painkillers known as endorphins. It is claimed that fifteen to twenty minutes' use of a TENS machine can overcome the pain for up to twelve hours depending on the problem, and that three out of four sufferers find it helpful. It seems to be used more and more these days in the treatment of back pain and to help pregnant women cope with labour pains.

Isobel has tried and tested quite a few physiotherapy treatments with nothing but praise as a result.

> I've had ice-packs on each ankle, and knees and hands, for about twenty minutes at a time. The coldness numbs the joint and therefore you get more freedom of movement and less pain. Remarkably I find that the effects last about four or five hours. After three weeks of this treatment I found that the effects lasted even longer.
>
> When you have arthritis, you have a fear of movement itself. The ice takes away the fear and a lot of the pain.

Isobel also found infra-red lamps directed at both shoulders helpful, warm and soothing; she describes Faradic footbaths as 'wonderful', as are the transcutaenous nerve stimulators, and she's pleased with the exercise programme devised for her.

Exercises should be done as often as you can without straining or causing discomfort (see the section on Exercise, page 82). It's best if you can follow a simple exercise routine twice a day. Says Isobel:

> I do them as best I can. I'm determined to be as fit as I can for a possible shoulder then knee replacement operation. Part of my routine is moving my feet up and down. Lifting my thigh up and holding for a minute, pretending I'm playing an imaginary piano with my fingers, clenching my fists as much as I am able, touching the tip of each finger with the tip of my thumb. You can feel muscles being worked – although I don't do exercises if I'm in severe pain or the inflammation is bad.

Other home exercises that may be helpful to you and which are sometimes recommended by physiotherapists include:

- **For hands**: place your hands flat on a table with your palms down and wrists still. Now move your hands from one side to the other.
- **For elbows:** tuck your elbows into your side, then while trying to keep them as still as possible, swivel the palms of your hands first upwards then downwards.
- **For shoulders:** put your hands on your shoulders then try to make circles with your elbows.
- **For ankles:** pull your ankles up towards you then point your toes away from you. And for the more adventurous, try picking up a pen or pencil from the floor with your toes.
- **For knees:** keeping your leg stiff, try to lift it off the bed without bending it and at the same time keeping your ankles at a right angle. Also, sitting in an upright chair, lift your feet about two inches off the floor.

There are of course dozens more exercise routines that can be practised easily at home.

Proper instructions on how to use your joints to avoid straining them can do much to help prevent deformities. So, in addition to administering pain-relieving treatment, a physiotherapist will plan exercises for you so that you can keep your muscles moving, naturally leading to greater mobility. Stiff joints just get more stiff if they're not used regularly, and when you have a painful joint, the natural tendency is to avoid using it.

Before doing any exercises at home, you may find it helpful to relieve any pain or muscle stiffness by first applying a hot water bottle or packet of frozen peas to affected areas. But if you do, be careful that the coldness hasn't numbed your joint to such an extent that you over-do the exercises without realising.

Looking after your joints isn't just a question of exercising regularly. You need to care for them on a day-to-day basis, for example, by using *both* your hands when you need to lift something. And stop carrying a heavy handbag filled with clutter that you never need and don't even know is in there! Think about ways you can avoid strain.

If you've never visited a physiotherapist you can ask your GP to refer you to a clinic attached to a hospital. By the way, some areas provide community physiotherapists to visit people at home, or you can get in touch with a private physiotherapist by contacting the Chartered Society of Physiotherapy (for address, see page 100).

In some regions hydrotherapy is offered as part of hospital physiotherapy. Hydrotherapy is basically physiotherapy exercises in water, usually in a specially heated pool.

Many arthritis sufferers tell me that they find this particularly helpful and even describe it as superb. They enjoy the warmth and soothing quality of the water. Also buoyancy allows you to move stiff joints more freely as it helps overcome gravity and this weightlessness means that the range of movement in an affected joint is much greater than when it is out of water.

Winifred, now sixty-two, has suffered from rheumatoid arthritis since she was in her early thirties. She's found anti-inflammatory drugs upset her stomach and despite being on steroids she feels as if she's 'getting nowhere'. For her, hydrotherapy has been a gift.

> It's one kind of treatment I actually look forward to. It loosens me up so much I can even walk more easily when I come out of the water. There are exercises that I find almost impossible when I'm out of the water but when I'm in it I can do them with ease and without putting any strain on my joints.
>
> Hydrotherapy is such a pleasant experience. The weightlessness helps you exercise and the warmth has a very soothing quality. It's so relaxing. It makes me feel so much better in myself and even helps me sleep well at night. As far as I'm concerned it's one of the best therapies there is and it doesn't cause any side-effects which is a bonus in itself!

For some people hydrotherapy can be tiring. Nevertheless the useful thing about it is that you can learn the special exercises and repeat them at your own pace and leisure in a local swimming pool. But make sure the pool is well heated. Warmth is needed to relax muscles and facilitate movement – there's not many of us who can relax and shiver at the same time. Fortunately, these days the water in public swimming pools is usually kept at a constant temperature of around 30°C.

Many sufferers also find that swimming is the one form of exercise they can do that aids their mobility without causing extra pain and damaged joints respond quite well to gentle stretching exercises done in water. Swimming is also a good way of looking after joints not affected by arthritis.

More and more local swimming pools offer 'quiet adult swim' sessions at off-peak times. These sessions are extremely useful for anyone wanting to try water exercises (bear in mind that you don't have to able to swim to do exercises in water) or to swim at a nice relaxed pace – although judging from the numbers and buzz of conversation at my local pool during these quiet adult swim sessions, more chatting than swimming goes on!

If you do find you're keen on swimming, there's also an Association for Swimming Therapy which could help you meet other swimmers. For address, see page 100. If you don't like going to swimming pools, your physiotherapist may be able to recommend simple stretching exercises that you could do at home in a warm bath.

Reducing stress on joints can be helpful not just by strengthening surrounding muscles but by resting the joints too. Splinting may sometimes be advised in order to rest inflamed joints, especially hands, wrists and knees, and to correct any possible deformities. 'Working' or dynamic splints (splints with moving parts) can help support wrists, for example, so a sufferer can carry out tasks around the home. In some areas these splints will be made by a physiotherapist, in others by an occupational therapist.

Splints can be used to ease pain, and help reduce swelling and inflammation; to try to re-align or prevent a deformity; to support or protect when muscles around a joint are weak and to act as an aid to healing after surgery. Dynamic splints can also help by stopping a joint moving unnecessarily or by giving additional support to a weak joint.

Usually, splints are not meant for constant use. Your therapist will decide which type is most suitable for you and for how long it should be worn. Whatever you do, don't try to make any DIY splints, leave it to the experts.

OCCUPATIONAL THERAPY

Some people have been known to panic, or even feel slightly insulted, if you recommend that they see an occupational therapist. But believe me, occupational therapy isn't all the fluffy toy-making and basket-weaving some people might think it is. These therapists are key people in the treatment and long-term management of arthritis.

The aims of occupational therapy are to help reduce pain. An important aspect of an occupational therapist's role is educating and encouraging a sufferer to manage any problems that arise by identifying both strengths and weaknesses, by building on what you can do and working out ways round what you can't. Occupational therapists are keen to help you reach and maintain as much independence as possible.

Your GP can put you in touch with an occupational therapist, or you could be referred to one as part of hospital treatment, to advise you on all manner of equipment to help you cope with day-to-day life. A therapist can look at your home or workplace and immediately advise you on ways of making life easier. Together you can tackle a particular problem and work out how to adapt to the limitations placed on you by arthritis. An occupational therapist will talk to you about how you're coping and will listen to your problems.

A complaint of some occupational therapists is often that they find people reluctant to take advice at the onset of rheumatic disease. Frequently, sufferers do not seek help until their arthritis has become so bad they are desperate for help. Yet, some occupational therapists (though not all) believe that 'joint preservation' is effective in preventing long-term joint damage.

Joint preservation involves thinking about how to look after and protect your joints even when your arthritis is just beginning or if you haven't had a flare-up for a while. It means establishing simple and efficient ways of doing things – for example, turning on to your side before rolling out of bed instead of putting your legs on to the floor then trying to drag the rest of your body along behind.

Joints ought to be used in the most efficient way possible, conserving your energy. If you have difficulty sitting down on to and getting up from the toilet, then an occupational therapist can advise you on having a raised toilet seat fitted. He or she can also determine precisely what the correct height should be. Don't struggle to pull yourself up by reaching out for a nearby radiator – not only does the stretching and pulling action put a strain on your joints but you could burn yourself or even pull the radiator away from the wall! Doing things awkwardly causes extra problems – hips and knees can be spared so much strain through a properly fitted raised toilet seat. And anyway, radiators weren't designed for acrobatics!

Many sufferers find a good soak in a hot bath eases their arthritis. But so often it is such hard work getting in and out of the bath, that the good work done by the relaxing soak is immediately undone. If you can afford it, try to have a walk-in shower installed. These are so much easier for you to manoeuvre in and out of – and after a while you'll probably enjoy a hot, invigorating shower as much as a long, hot bath. If you can't afford a shower, ask your occupational therapist to suggest other ways of cheaply modifying your bathroom.

Joint preservation also means not straining your finger joints by picking up too many heavy things, too many small things at once, or struggling with bottle and jar tops. Opening packs of tablets or medicine bottles with childproof 'press and turn' lids, or the flip-top type with arrows that you have to align, becomes a constant battle of will for many arthritis sufferers. When rheumatologists at a Manchester hospital asked two hundred elderly or arthritic patients to open twelve drug containers, three-quarters of them had difficulty doing so. A quarter said they couldn't get at the contents of three containers at all! So do bear in mind that medicine bottles with non-childproof tops can be obtained from the chemist.

Apparently, many arthritis sufferers find jar openers perfectly acceptable yet they're reluctant to have tap-turners fitted or to enlarge their door knobs to prevent unnecessary strain on wrist joints. If you consider how many times taps are turned on and off and doors are opened and closed in the course of a week, these preventative measures are vital.

Energy preservation is another simple but important piece of advice constantly given by occupational therapists and about which there seems to be agreement within the profession. Fatigue is a symptom of arthritis and this is true for all the different types, in particular the more severe forms. Also just coping with arthritis can drain your energy. If the disease is going through an active phase you can be weak so there's absolutely no point in using up energy that could have been saved.

Planning your routines can help. If you do your washing on a Monday morning, you don't need to iron it and put it all away the same day. If you know you need to go shopping on a Thursday, then try to rest on Wednesdays. If you are tired in the early evening and never seem to be in the mood for cooking then, either take your main meal in the middle of the day or at least prepare the vegetables earlier when you have more energy. You could even cook a casserole in the morning which could simply be reheated in the evening.

Find out what equipment can help you carry out simple jobs in half the time it would take you otherwise. Jobs like opening tins, peeling potatoes, drawing curtains, pulling down blinds, putting on tights – the list is endless. One simple adjustment, which saves fiddling around with a door key for ages, is to have the rounded end made bigger. A simple idea but so useful.

With hips and knees affected by osteoarthritis, bending can be particularly difficult and there is a wide variety of aids available to make life easier in that respect – for instance, special long-handled 'pick-up sticks' or extra-long shoe horns.

Then there are velcro fastenings for clothes instead of buttons and zips (provided the strip which pulls away from the grip part of the Velcro is long enough to pull without difficulty), plus various other aids to dressing. One of the most useful pieces of equipment is a dressing stick. This is usually a 15-inch piece of dowel, half an inch in diameter. It has a rubber thimble at one end and a cup hook screwed into the other end. It's wonderful for pulling cardigans on over shoulders, putting on underwear, drawing back curtains and many, many more jobs. Ask your occupational therapist about how you can get one. Some clinics make them on site.

My advice is, if you're offered a hospital appointment or a home assessment with an occupational therapist then seize the opportunity. There's nothing to be gained by being obstinate about accepting help. You can ask their advice about any particular problem that needs a practical solution. You'll be amazed at what they can come up with.

As I said earlier, your GP can put you in touch with an occupational therapist, or you can contact one direct by phoning your local social services department. You can also contact the College of Occupational Therapists for a private practice register. Occupational therapists who have completed a three- or four-year training course use the letters DipCOT after their name, as well as SROT if they select to go on to the state register.

Arthritis Care and the Disabled Living Foundation are also invaluable sources of information for you, make sure you use their services. For addresses and telephone numbers, see pages 99, 100. Arthritis Care runs a small grants scheme and may be able to help if there is a piece of equipment you need but cannot afford. Write to them for an application form or just if you'd like to know more about it. The Disabled Living Foundation has an equipment centre which demonstrates a large range of equipment. It has functional areas to show kitchen, bathroom and toilet aids and adaptations. Other sections include clothing and footwear.

So, get help sooner rather than later. Just because you accept help doesn't mean you aren't in control of your life. One occupational therapist told me, the worse and most upsetting thing an arthritis sufferer can say to her is, 'I'm managing.' You may be managing, but at what expense to your joints?

Jane, a forty-four-year-old housewife, has found that

occupational therapy has been of great value to her and made quite a difference to her life. A former hairdresser, she has rheumatoid arthritis and was forced to give up work because the disease affected her feet, knees, hands and elbows so severely.

> My feet have been very badly affected. I felt as if I were walking on pebbles. I had surgery to try to improve the situation, including pins being put into my toes to straighten them.
>
> Following surgery I was on crutches for several months and it was about a year before I could walk properly again. It was such a breakthough to walk without pain. My feet are by no means normal looking but they are marvellous to what they were. I still can't wear ordinary shoes but I adapt and wear boots.

Jane has also had surgery on her hands and wrists but she is unable to bend her right hand at all. With such restraints on her mobility she has found occupational therapy of immense value.

> To be honest, my occupational therapist is so helpful that I ring her whenever I have a problem because of my joints and ask her advice.
>
> I now know that I have to pace myself. I accept what I can and can't do. I have help from a home-carer. She comes to my home twice a week for two hours. This is so helpful. She does all the ironing and peels enough vegetables for a few days at a time, which I then put in the fridge. One thing I just can't do is peel vegetables.

Jane's home has been organised to erase obstacles from her day-to-day life. Her occupational therapist suggested more efficient ways of coping, even down to advice on what to wear.

My therapist highlighted the things I could do that I wouldn't have thought of otherwise. Before buying clothes I think about how easy or difficult they are going to be to wear. I never buy anything that has lots of buttons or only does up at the back.

I've got an electric can opener. I have a special knife with its handle at a right angle to the blade. I use that for everything, including opening cereal packets and packets of washing powder.

My oven is now at a different level, it's just below waist height. All my kitchen cupboards have been lowered. I have a dishwasher which I find wonderful to use. It means I can load the dishes myself. All my kitchen cupboards have been lowered, which makes things much easier. I have a washing machine with touch button control and I use a potato masher to open it.

My bed has been raised. I'm about five feet five inches tall and the bed is at the same height as the top of my leg. This makes my life so much easier in the morning when I tend to be very stiff. Getting into bed at night has been made easier, too.

My toilet seat has also been raised. I have a walk-in shower. This is very useful because it saves me struggling to get in and out of the bath.

All these adaptations have made such a difference to me. I immediately notice how much more awkward things are if I visit someone else's house.

Instead of being reluctant to accept help, Jane embraced it – and has found life much easier to cope with because of it.

For the last year or so I also have help from a lady who is part of a local Crossroads scheme. She comes for three hours on a Monday when she cleans the upstairs, changes the beds, does the toilet and bathroom. That way I only have the downstairs to worry about.

It puts my mind at rest so much. I used to find that when I didn't feel well it made me feel even worse if the place was in a mess. And some days I do feel so weary, although at the moment I feel very good and I haven't had any flare-ups for a while.

If I can do a certain amount myself I don't feel guilty about not being able to do anything. By accepting help, I feel much better and I still feel as if I am in control of my life because I organise what needs to be done. It really is worthwhile finding out about the help you can get.

SELF-HELP TREATMENT

You know, it's surprising just how much people are able to do to help themselves. For some, this can simply mean finding a person they can talk to honestly about the way they feel. For others, learning to perfect something as straightforward and useful as relaxation techniques can be as beneficial as anything else.

Once arthritis has been diagnosed, many sufferers like to control their own pain without constantly 'bothering' their doctor or find that for managing mild to moderate pain they are happy to buy products over the counter. It's been suggested that some arthritis sufferers never even go to see their doctor or seek any help at all. These people should come to no harm providing they are not taking painkillers every day. If such medicines are needed all or most of the time, it is much wiser to see your doctor.

For mild cases of arthritis you may find aspirin a useful pain-reliever. Aspirin can be bought over the counter in pharmacies and supermarkets under own brand names or many trade names such as Aspro or Solmin. It's effective against the pain of arthritis as well as inflammation, but as I have said before (see page 49) it can irritate the stomach and cause indigestion, as well as aggravating stomach ulcers.

Ibuprofen (Nurofen, Inoven) is another popular over-the-counter medicine (see page 49). When people have taken it they find it gentler on the stomach than aspirin even though it works in similar ways. Nevertheless, you still shouldn't take it if you have a stomach ulcer, or are allergic to aspirin. It may also cause asthma in those prone to it.

Paracetamol can be used when aspirin isn't suitable, although it doesn't reduce inflammation. Like aspirin, paracetamol is widely available under own brand names or trade names such as Panadol or Paraclear. Other painkillers contain mixtures of paracetamol and codeine, such as

Solpadeine, or paracetamol, aspirin and codeine in the case of Veganin, which can be useful in controlling rheumatic pain.

If you take painkillers, don't mix and match them. Always consult your doctor or pharmacist before taking an over-the-counter medicine if you are already taking medication or have a medical condition. If you are taking one type of analgesic don't take another within four hours – overdoses can be dangerous. Never exceed the stated dose and follow directions on the packet very carefully. Taking a lot of medicine in one go does not mean it will work more efficiently or more speedily, and it can be harmful.

Having given you those warnings, I can also give you a small piece of advice. If you know that something is going to be painful but you need to get it done, – for example, shopping or going to the bank – then taking a painkiller an hour before you go can make the trip that much easier. Remember that tablets or capsules can stick in your throat, so do swallow them with plenty of water and always while you're sitting or standing up.

Arthritis sufferers tell me that cold treatments are beneficial. The ubiquitous packet of frozen peas is a popular way of numbing a painful area, but do protect your skin by keeping a damp cloth or flannel between you and the packet. Rubbing the affected area with ice cubes, similarly wrapped, can also be helpful. Cold treatment can be useful in easing hot, swollen joints, but be careful not to move the affected joint too much afterwards because cold can numb pain and you may put strain on your joint without realising.

Other sufferers prefer heat treatment. Warmth from a hot bath or shower, careful use of an electric blanket or heat applied by a hot water bottle (wrapped in a dry or damp towel to prevent burning your skin) are simple, inexpensive methods – although they are not to be recommended for a very inflamed (that is, a swollen, hot and and tender) joint, because extra heat may make the inflammation even worse. Don't use heat treatments when you are tired either, because you could fall asleep and then burn your skin.

Warmth is especially useful if you have aching or stiff joints and muscles. It could be beneficial first thing in the morning if you find your stiffness worse then. You needn't use heat treatment for more than twenty minutes and keep an eye on your skin during and after. Skin shouldn't be bright red – that means you've either had too much warmth or you've been cooking too long!

Remember that you shouldn't use heat or cold treatments on your arthritic joints if you have poor circulation in your hands or feet, if you have any numbness, or if your skin isn't as sensitive as normal, in case you scald yourself without realising. And, if you have heart problems, check first with your doctor. For example, a hot bath – though beneficial – can strain a weak heart.

Widely available rubs and liniments can ease rheumatic pain and arthritis and provide welcome temporary relief. Rubbing in a cream or spraying the affected area can work by a process called counter-irritation, superficial irritation of the skin to relieve a deep-seated type of pain.

There are many rubs and liniments on the market including Algipan Rub and Spray, Bengue's Balsam, Boots Warming Pain Relief Spray, Boots Icy-Gel Muscle Rub, Boots Pain Relieving Balm, the Deep Heat range of products (especially Deep Heat Intensive Therapy and Deep Heat Deep Freeze Cold Gel), Massage Balm, Menthol and Wintergreen Rub, PR Freeze Spray, PR Heat Spray, and the Radian-B Range.

ARTHRITIS, DIET, SUPPLEMENTS AND LUCKY CHARMS

In my opinion, food on its own doesn't make a person healthy – what's important is eating a balanced diet. So if you suffer from arthritis and have wondered whether a special diet might allow you to move with ease and have nights without pain, but have also wondered whether the suggested link between diet and and arthritis is just another fashionable fad, I wouldn't blame you for one minute for being confused. The evidence for this link provokes argument, claims, counter-claims and confusion even in the medical profession.

There seems to be no consensus of opinion on what should or shouldn't be eaten and there's certainly not enough space in this book to devote pages to the controversy surrounding diet and arthritis. But I'll try to guide you in what I hope is the right direction. Briefly, some specialists believe that one of the many causes of arthritis may be a deficiency of vitamins or minerals, particularly iron, calcium, zinc or selenium; or it may be an allergy to food additives and preservatives, and all manner of other basic foodstuffs, from dairy products to cereal. Consequently they advise a high protein diet of fish, fresh vegetables and rice to relieve symptoms. But as I've said, opinion is divided even among doctors who agree that careful diet can ease symptoms. Some proponents say that steak, eggs and cheese should be eaten, others argue the opposite.

To add to the confusion there seems to be some evidence that cutting out food almost altogether can bring relief. This, of course, is not to be recommended as the 'benefits' are not at all long-lasting and symptoms tend to return once you start eating normally again. It's thought that any improvement the sufferer may notice could be linked to an alteration in the way the immune system works, plus the body's production of other inflammation-causing substances from food is thought to be reduced, too.

There are people who completely reject the idea that what you eat can ease your pain, but perhaps this is being too narrow-minded as some things do seem to work for some people.

Without doubt, there is one form of arthritis that *does* respond to diet and that's gout – long thought of as the result of too much good food and good wine. Through no fault of their own, people with gout need to be careful about what they eat and drink. As I've already explained in an earlier section of the book (see page 33), gout is caused by

higher than normal levels of uric acid, which is manufac-
tured from purines in food. If you have too much purine in
your diet levels of uric acid will be increased and this is likely
to spur an attack.

Alcohol can also change blood uric acid levels, so drink
only a moderate amount – the pain of another attack of gout
surely isn't worth risking. Anyone prone to gout would be
sensible to avoid foods high in purines such as liver, bacon,
kidneys, sweetbreads, fish roe, anchovies, herrings, mack-
erel, mussels, sardines, yeast extracts (e.g. Marmite), yeast
and beers. Those low in purine are tea, coffee, cereal, cheese,
eggs and milk. You should also avoid over-eating in general.

Some sufferers have read that Eskimos who eat high
quantities of oily fish seem to suffer fewer diseases such as
cancer, arthritis and coronary heart diseases, and thousands
of people these days seem very keen on religiously swallow-
ing oil supplements. Take a look at pharmacy and health-
food shop shelves bulging with cod liver oil (both capsules
and liquid form) and capsules of fish oil, halibut oil, salmon
oil, evening primrose oil, even fish oil and primrose oil
combined, or the reverse combination of evening primrose
oil and fish oil! You'll see what I mean.

However, it is indeed now recognised that diets low in
saturated fats, or that include fish oil or primrose oil which
contain polyunsaturated fatty acids, may be beneficial in
arthritis. According to the ARC (the Arthritis and Rheumatism Council) these fatty acids are used by the body to
make chemicals which are less inflammatory than those
made from fats in a diet without them. Therefore fish oils
and evening primrose oil can have a mild anti-inflammatory
effect. A Scottish study has also revealed that taking fish oil
regularly for at least three months may mean that you need
fewer painkillers, or even none at all, as well as having fewer
tender and swollen joints.

If you want to try fish oil or evening primrose then take
one or the other. There's no point taking both. You also
have to be aware that once you start taking them, you'll

need to carry on because any benefits seem to be lost once you stop.

Some of my readers tell me that they 'oil their joints'! While this is not how it works, the benefits are appreciated by many sufferers!

George, a seventy-nine-year-old retired electrical engineer, insists that cod liver oil supplements and fishy changes in his diet have eased the symptoms of rheumatoid arthritis.

> Stiffness and a toothache-like pain in my shoulders meant I couldn't sleep. In the morning, stiffness was even worse. My legs would be almost seized up and at times I couldn't get out of bed. I couldn't open my hands in the morning without putting them under cold running water for quite a while first.
>
> I've never liked taking tablets and when I'd read that diet might be able to help arthritis I decided anything was worth a try. I didn't see that at my age I had much to lose. I also didn't see that at my age I should give in to arthritis either. I don't eat any meat or chicken. I eat oily fish, such as mackerel, tuna, salmon or herring, nearly every day as well as taking the recommended dose of cod liver oil tablets. It may be hard to believe but I honestly noticed a difference within a month.
>
> Now a few months later, the stiffness isn't nearly as bad and the pain has eased so much I can manage without taking painkillers, which I couldn't before. I can sleep at night, instead of waking every hour and then being too tired to get up in the morning. I can also drive again, do housework and take my dog for a walk. Simple things, but things that mean a lot to me.

Many sufferers like George believe wholeheartedly that diet modifications and fish oil supplements do help. Others swear by a selenium supplement mixed with vitamins A, C and E (see page 79), while others recommend olive oil, soya milk, brewers' yeast, cider vinegar in warm water first thing in the morning, or eating molasses. Even a substance known as propolis, a sticky resin derived from trees and used by bees to seal cracks in the hive and keep it clear of germs, is said to help arthritis. Yet hard evidence proving that diet really *does* have a significant effect on arthritis is thin on the ground. That doesn't mean doctors don't take it seriously, however. Many are now advocating low-fat diets which cut out red meat, full-fat milk and butter (even confectionery made with butter), and promote 'oily' fish or vegetable oil, to help reduce the need for painkillers and anti-inflammatory drugs.

Ruth, a thirty-three-year-old secretary, also suffering from rheumatoid arthritis, has found relief by changing her diet drastically and following a 'sensible' eating plan.

> I first had rheumatoid arthritis when I was twelve years old. It appeared in my toe then in my knees. It was painful but I was able to carry on with my life normally and with my schooling.
>
> When I was about twenty-six, I began to get flare-ups of the disease that would put me out of action. It also then affected my back and I couldn't move an inch without excruciating pain.
>
> After that it spread into virtually all my joints and was kept under control with anti-inflammatory drugs. But the flare-ups increased in severity. One was so excruciatingly painful that I couldn't even bear to have my bed sheets touch me. The only way to avoid this was having a cage in my bed to keep them away from me. My hands, knees and feet would be the worst affected. They'd be huge, swollen and so hot. I'd wrap them in ice-cold towels to try to get rid of the heat.

A friend of Ruth's suggested she contact the Arthritic Association – an association which believes in the use of 'natural' methods of treatment. These include homoeopathic remedies, sensible eating and, in some cases, massage therapy.

> I was in such a state four years ago. I was only twenty-nine years old. I'd taken lots of anti-inflammatory drugs and even steroids for a short while. Yet I was in such pain I would have tried anything.
>
> I followed the dietary advice given by the Arthritic Association – a sensible wholefood eating plan. I'm supposed to eat an abundance of fresh, raw fruit and vegetables, lots of pulses, grains, whole-meal pasta, for example. I can eat chicken, cheese, nuts and fish – which I hate – but I have to avoid red meat, refined, processed and canned foods.
>
> I was open-minded about the effects the diet might have. I used to eat a lot of junk food and lots of sweets. I also drank lots of tea and coffee. For the first two weeks I felt very lethargic. I'm sure that was because I'd suddenly cut out all that tea and coffee.

Slowly and surely over the next few months Ruth's arthritis began to improve. From being totally out of action because of terrible pain and swelling four years ago, she's now working again.

> Changing my diet has helped me tremendously. My general health has improved and my energy levels have definitely increased. I've found my diet keeps the inflammation down as well as the pain. I don't take any medication now – not even for a headache. Sometimes I have pain in my joints but only when I indulge myself and cheat on the diet.
>
> I recognise that in certain cases drugs are helpful but in my own case, and through my own personal

choice, I felt that at my age if I could manage then I would.

Four years ago I was in such a bad state. Now I'm able to work part-time and hope to go back to full-time soon. I think if you can help yourself by diet then it's worth a try. It's a natural way to try to improve your health.

These days Ruth considers what she's eating before she eats it – so much so that healthy eating has become second nature and she craves salads the way some people crave chocolate.

I never used to think about what I ate. I'd eat whatever I fancied. Now I do think carefully about what I eat. The diet has really turned the tables on my eating habits – although I do admit I miss the cream cakes!

Changing her diet does seem to have worked for Ruth, but Bev, a thirty-one-year-old mother of three who has rheumatoid arthritis, hasn't found that careful diet and supplements alter her symptoms at all. She has suffered for thirteen years and her feet, ankles, knees, hands and elbows have been particularly affected. She believes she eats a healthy diet anyway, with lots of fresh fruit and vegetables and not a lot of red meat, and she has tried oil supplements.

I took evening primrose oil for about two years and there was no change in the inflammation. I don't know whether I took a big enough dose. But I've also tried cod liver oil, halibut liver oil and fish oil supplements and none of them made any difference.

If you have mild symptoms perhaps it might help you. As far as I'm concerned I think it's too simple a remedy and that the answer to arthritis is much more complicated than that.

I have to say that, in general, much more information and research is needed about arthritis and diet. The clear-cut evidence isn't as exciting as many of the claims. Yet some sufferers do find that just giving up something – say, wheat products – seems to help their arthritis.

Gary, the trainee surveyor who talked about his rheumatoid arthritis earlier in the book, is an example of someone who noticed that certain things in his diet made his joint stiffness worse. He has repeatedly found that eating lots of chocolate and drinking more than the odd glass of wine or pint of beer does aggravate his symptoms so he now avoids too much of either.

> When I was about nineteen I used to drink more beer than I do now. At the time I drank, the pain seemed to subside so that encouraged me to carry on. I would have perhaps four pints quite often because it helped me get to sleep. But it wasn't worth it because the pain and stiffness was much worse the next day.
>
> I don't drink that often now because of the effects alcohol has but if we go to a party or something and I might have four pints, I do still notice quite a difference the next day.
>
> Normally I get up at about six-thirty in the morning and I can manage to move around quite well. If I've had a drink the night before it takes me ages to get going – sometimes it's as late as midday.

If you find that a particular food or drink aggravates your arthritis then I see no harm in avoiding that foodstuff, providing you are still getting all the nutrients you require. What I am concerned about is that if you're in constant pain because of arthritis you could clutch at straws in an attempt to rid yourself of that pain and thus upset your diet. Having said that, there are doctors who feel that special diets can result in less pain and fewer side-effects than perhaps some conventional methods of treatment.

The problem with trying to prove that diet helps ease arthritis is that mind over matter could play a part. A patient may so desperately want to feel better that his or her imagination could influence any feeling of improvement due to cutting out, say, flour, or cereals, or dairy products. Also, the fact that a special diet may result in a patient losing some weight can interfere with research, as weight loss itself, especially if a sufferer is overweight, can sometimes ease pain (see page 52). And the trouble with arthritis, as any sufferer will tell you, is that you get good days and bad days. So a natural good spell, or just going into remission, could also cause a blip in any research results.

What you have to remember is that some things work for some people and healthy, nutritionally balanced meals with fresh fruit and vegetables will usually do more good than harm.

It doesn't take much common sense to work out that eating a balanced diet – with moderation as well as variety in all things – is a fundamental aid to basic good health. Fresh fruit and vegetables are excellent sources for topping up your daily vitamin levels. Fish, meat and poultry provide the essential protein you need, but choose lean cuts of meat, eat chicken without the skin, and always grill or bake instead of frying. You should try to eat fish or poultry instead of meat two or three times a week. Milk, eggs, cheese, oily fish and nuts also contain healthy vitamins, minerals, proteins and other essential nutrients.

By following a sensible eating plan, particularly cutting down on saturated fats (often hidden in many foods like pies, sausage rolls, pasties, cakes and biscuits) you'll probably find you'll lose weight. And as I've said before, being overweight doesn't do arthritis sufferers any favours. If you're overweight you are more likely to develop osteoarthritis, for instance, because of the extra pressure on your hips and knees. Losing weight thus reduces mechanical strain on the weight-bearing joints.

Research supported by the American National Institute of Health claims that reducing your weight slightly is a good way to prevent osteoarthritis and even the need for a joint replacement later in life. Women tend to put on weight as they get older, but in the survey when women of average height lost eleven pounds in weight over twelve years their chances of developing the disease were cut in half! However, the arthritis is not caused simply because these joints have to carry excess weight. Since people who are overweight also seem to be more at risk of getting osteoarthritis in their fingers and hands.

Losing weight, with your doctor's approval, will also affect your general sense of well-being and hopefully you won't feel so sluggish.

There is still little evidence to convince all the medical profession that extra vitamins, minerals or trace elements are beneficial in the treatment of arthritis. But some people like to feel that they have some control over their 'treatment' and prefer to try supplements all the same.

One trace element proving popular in the last few years with people suffering from arthritis is selenium. It's called a trace element because the amount needed to keep us healthy is so tiny – though none the less essential. Some research has shown that two minerals, selenium and zinc, have a helpful effect on our immune system and so it's thought that selenium could help relieve arthritis. To be effective it is recommended to be taken with Vitamin E. Vitamins A and C are also thought to increase its benefits.

Green-lipped mussel extract (a native of New Zealand) is another supplement that hit the headlines because of its claimed anti-inflammatory properties. The treatment involves taking up to three to five capsules, or one or two tablets, of the extract every day, depending on the strength you buy. They can be bought in health shops and chemists under the brand names of Seatone or Musseltone and will cost you roughly between five pounds and ten pounds for a month's supply depending on the brand, the strength you buy and the quantity you take.

According to ARC, it appears to do no harm, although

there's no satisfactory evidence that it improves or 'cures' arthritis. You pays your money and you takes your choice! To be on the safe side you shouldn't take mussel extract if you're allergic to seafood.

Royal jelly, it is claimed, is a good source of vitamins, minerals and amino acids as in nature it's fed exclusively to the queen bee so that she can live a long and fertile life. It's said to contain ninety-six nutrients and enzymes in all. As far as I'm concerned this gives some people a 'fairytale' reason for taking it, believing that it must 'do you good'. That alone is not convincing enough for me.

Herbal remedies do seem to be increasing in popularity these days. But please be aware that just because a remedy has been used for hundreds of years, or just because it's 'natural' it's not necessarily OK. 'Natural' doesn't automatically mean 'harmless' or 'without side-effects', such as irritability or sleeplessness, for example.

Ginseng, also called the 'Root of Life', is the root of a plant that has been used in the Far East for more than five thousand years. It's said to contain beneficial organic acids, vitamins, minerals, enzymes and amino acids which are thought to increase energy and general zest for life. But it's also thought to increase blood pressure – so caution is necessary in those known to be hypertensive.

Potter's, Heath and Heather, and Gerard herbal products are popular and are available from health shops and some chemists. Potter's have a remedy called 'Tabritis' for the symptomatic relief of rheumatic pain and stiffness. Gerard herbal remedies include Kelp, also for the symptomatic relief of rheumatic pain. Heath and Heather make Celery Seed tablets and Rheumatic Pain tablets.

The herbal remedies available from chemists, health shops and even supermarkets may be helpful for minor problems, but, if your symptoms are persistent or more severe, it is best – so as to avoid quacks – to consult a registered medical herbalist (who will have the letters MNIMH or FNIMH after their name) for a full assessment and tailormade prescription. Two people with apparently the same symptoms may be given quite different prescriptions as the herbalist takes so many factors into account. Professional herbalists (a lot of people aren't even aware of their existence) are trained to use many of the same diagnostic methods as doctors and to refer people for x-rays and other specialist investigations or treatment, if necessary. For more information about herbal medicine contact the National Institute of Medical Herbalists (see page 101).

Take a walk along any high street on a Saturday afternoon and I'm sure you'll spot dozens of people wearing copper bracelets. They're almost seen as lucky charms to ward off disease. I don't think there's any real evidence they do any good, but then I'm sure they don't do any harm either – apart from sometimes leaving a green stain on the skin.

I imagine that some people wear them because they think they will absorb copper through their skin and that this will help their arthritis in some way. In fact, according to ARC, recent work has shown that people with rheumatoid arthritis usually have a higher than normal level of copper anyway, so it doesn't look as if they need any more.

Copper bracelets aren't a magic cure. I suppose if some sufferers believe that their bracelets do some good, then it's all a matter of choice – and some people are so convinced of this, I wouldn't like to persuade them to take them off!

Provided you have discussed the idea fully with your own doctor then making changes to your diet or taking supplements may help you. Even if someone you know has been helped by, for example, taking evening primrose oil for six months to help alleviate the symptoms of rheumatoid arthritis, don't expect a miracle cure. You could well be disappointed if you do.

EXERCISE – AND REST

A recent national survey by the Sports Council and the Health Education Authority has revealed that three-quarters of all adults don't take enough exercise. Yet exercise keeps you in trim, increases your stamina, helps maintain a healthy heart and is a good means of relieving stress. It isn't just important for helping your arthritis, therefore, it's good for your general health, too.

When you have arthritis your joints need to be looked after properly to help keep discomfort at a minimum and stop even more damage. One report has shown that when more than one hundred people with arthritic knees followed an exercise programme for eight weeks their general health improved and their arthritis didn't seem to bother them as much. Exercise aids mobility, is thought to reduce pain and protects your joints by keeping the muscles strong.

Arthritis can make you feel fatigued very easily so when exercising think 'little and often' and take plenty of rest in between. Many sufferers have told me that they do what they can when they can. Even if your physiotherapist has suggested exercises for you to do regularly at home, do only what has been advised, don't over-do it and try not to make too many repetitive movements, particularly on a joint affected by arthritis. If you feel tired or in pain when you're walking or exercising then stop. An ache should not be harmful but real pain is telling you that the limit has been reached. Within this limit, it is important to keep as active and mobile as possible, interspersed with periods of rest, though try to avoid spending too long in the same position. And a word of warning – certainly don't try exercising when you may be going through a flare-up.

Contact sports are certainly not helpful to sufferers because the joints can be easily injured. A physiotherapist can advise you on what type of exercise would help you if you are unsure of how far you should push yourself. Gentle exercise such as swimming or ordinary walking at a nice relaxed pace shouldn't do you any harm. Walking is inexpensive and improves your heart function, blood circulation and lung capacity.

Aerobic exercise is thought to encourage the production of endorphins (the body's natural painkillers). It is this type of sustained exercise which really gets your heart and lungs working hard. Some experts think that endorphins could aid the reduction of inflammation in inflammatory diseases. No one knows whether this is so or not, but exercise can make you feel generally better.

It's helpful if you try to exercise at the time of day that's best for you. Perhaps this is when you are least stiff and have the most energy.

Don't push yourself beyond your own limitations just because you know of a fellow arthritis sufferer who exercises more than you do. Remember, the success of any exercise plan depends on whether you enjoy it in the first place. Treat it as pleasure not punishment. If you enjoy walking all year round, however, bear in mind that people with arthritis who move slowly do run a risk of hypothermia. You can lose heat without even realising it, so make sure you wear several layers of clothing – several layers are better than one thick one as they're more efficient at trapping heat. And don't stay outdoors too long in cold weather. Use a walking stick if you find it helps – this can stop too much pressure being put on an arthritic hip or knee.

Rest, in the form of a good night's sleep is important, too, particularly when your arthritis is active. Rest is crucial in lupus, for example, where fatigue is a common problem. If you find sleeping difficult, try learning some relaxation techniques, see page 84.

What's important to remember when you have arthritis is striking a balance between rest and exercise. Without exercise joints can stiffen and bones and muscles weaken. People who exercise regularly tend to have lower stress levels, more energy and consequently become more productive.

RELAXATION TECHNIQUES

Above, I've talked about the benefits of exercise, but I also believe you shouldn't put all your energy into filling spare time with exercises alone. Make time for relaxing!

Relaxation techniques are very useful in the self-help ways of coping with arthritis. Chronic pain can interrupt your sleeping pattern and it can also make you feel depressed and irritable – through no fault of your own. This type of pain can make you anxious which in turn makes you tense your muscles, tugging on the joints and adding to your discomfort. You can easily become trapped in a vicious circle of pain, then tension, then more pain. Relaxation helps you cope with pain and aids sleep.

Ann, who I've mentioned above, follows a simple and effective relaxation routine of tensing muscles and then relaxing them that's easy to remember. She finds it helps her break that cycle of pain and tension – physical relaxation cuts down on muscle tension and mental relaxation helps keep her calm.

> I tense my jaw muscles then let them go. By doing that you quickly feel the difference between a tense muscle and a relaxed one. I work my way down my body doing the tensing and relaxing very slowly.
>
> It's not always easy to concentrate and get the knack of it particularly if you're in a lot of pain. But I find it so relaxing I often use this technique if I wake in the night. I soon find it settles me down and I can fall asleep again.

It helps if you choose half an hour or so when you know you're unlikely to be disturbed. There's also little to be gained from trying to relax when you are very stiff or are in a lot of pain. Of course, once you are used to unwinding in this way, you can then use the technique to help you cope with that kind of pain. Another useful pointer when starting out is to try to have a bed or sofa to lie on and try to make sure the room you use is comfortably warm and peaceful.

It can take a while before you perfect the technique – you may even need to give it a go every day for a month. But once perfected you'll probably find it won't matter where you are. And you can spend as long as you think you need to relax totally.

You can learn to relax by resting with your arms and legs unfolded and uncrossed. Think about the way you are breathing and try to breathe slowly and regularly. Focus on your muscles and imagine that they are becoming very heavy. Or, as Ann says, concentrate on different parts of your body, working down from your head to your toes. When you release your muscles let them go as much as possible. It helps, too, if you take long, slow breaths and try to think about nothing else or, if you can't clear your mind, at least think of something pleasant!

POSITIVE THINKING

Adapting your life to take arthritis into account can present you with all sorts of problems and provoke a whole range of emotions. One younger sufferer told me that arthritis when you're young makes you grieve for the future. Peggy, who's in her eighties, told me simply, 'Arthritis makes you feel old.' But, despite her age she doesn't feel old when she has a good day.

Many older people seem to accept arthritis as an inevitable part of growing old. For younger sufferers, coming to terms with the disease can be much more traumatic and lead to feelings of bitterness about an active life that's been snatched away before it's properly begun.

Paul, a forty-year-old principal scientist, has suffered with arthritis for thirteen years. He's been diagnosed as having 'incomplete' Reiter's syndrome. 'I haven't had conjunctivitis or lower back problems. Yet my arthritis definitely seemed to follow on from a viral infection.'

His ankles, feet and toes, knees and hands have been particularly affected by severe pain and stiffness. He spent periods in hospital, tried anti-inflammatory to anti-malarial drugs, and had a synovectomy on his right knee, before he finally responded to 'gold' therapy (see page 00).

Paul can only describe his feelings at the onset of the disease as total panic and fright, followed by depression and anger.

> I was really frightened that my life was at an end. Frightened that my girlfriend Debbie, now my wife, would leave me. It was all too terrifying to begin to describe. I then got angry and took it out on other people. People close to me and even strangers.
>
> A couple of times I went out feeling sorry for myself. I had too much to drink and was abusive to people I didn't even know. It was shameful behaviour but that's how my own fear manifested itself.

Initially, Paul believes, being admitted to hospital is a frightening experience in itself.

> Seeing other people so much worse than you, especially seeing children with the disease is terrible.
>
> Emotionally, it was such a hell of a shock for me at the age of twenty-seven. I'd always associated arthritis with old age. I was lucky in one way that I was still a student doing postgraduate studies, at least I wasn't in industry then.
>
> Even so my confidence went. At that age you feel that nothing can touch you. Your life will be perfect but then suddenly you are hit by this strange ailment that stops you doing everything. That's when you begin to appreciate other people's problems. You're not immune from the horrendous things that can occur in life any more.

Embarrassment is another emotion Paul recalls: he found

it difficult to admit to friends that he couldn't carry on in the ways he'd always done before.

> Friends and I would meet at a pub for a drink. After a while they'd want to move on to a pub half a mile up a hill. I was just too embarrassed to tell them I couldn't walk properly and couldn't keep up with them. I'd rather struggle and be in pain than ask them to slow down.

Admitting you can't cope is hard for many people with arthritis, as is accepting other people's help or being forced to be dependent on others for the first time in their lives. And adapting to the restrictions arthritis can impose on your life is one of the most difficult aspects of coming to terms with the disease. Not just for the arthritis sufferer but for partners and families, too.

Paul's wife, Debbie, says:

> If I'm honest, I have to say I've found coping with Paul's disease hard at times. In the early days I was very frightened. At one stage he could barely move and I didn't know how I would cope if he didn't get better and became completely disabled. I knew I would probably have had to give up my career to look after him.
>
> Arthritis has affected our life together in all sorts of ways. We didn't get married for about five years after Paul first developed arthritis. There were no guarantees that he would get better. And again, being totally honest, that was partly because I was making sure I could cope if he was bad again. Your marriage vows are for better or worse. Usually people haven't experienced the 'worse' at that stage.
>
> It's also played a part in our decision not to have children because I know Paul feels he wouldn't be able to play with them the way he would want to, for example.

Sometimes I do feel selfish and I wonder why we have to put up with it and how different life would have been for us without arthritis.

Paul agrees that both partners have to adapt, not just the one with arthritis. He's found that having a stable and supportive relationship has helped him cope and motivates him to get as much out of life as he can. But having arthritis can make you feel tired and, naturally, edgy. Friends and family ought to make allowances, but it's not always as straightforward as that.

Because you look well people forget that you're not. I'm not inclined to point out that I can't do things. I can't run up the road. I can't do things around the house I'd like to do, not just in terms of DIY but housework too. I can put in effort for a certain time – but even walking up and down stairs can be a strain.

So I push myself too hard and physical activity affects me, particularly my knees. After wearing myself out I lose my temper and demand to know why people have expected me to do something – rather than remind them in the first place that I'm restricted in what I can do, even though I know when I do too much I'll be stiffer and in more pain than usual the next day.

Says Debbie:

I do forget when Paul looks so well and doesn't complain. I get angry with him too because he pushes himself far too hard at work just because he feels that his disability reflects on him as a person and on his ability to do his job. I can understand how he feels but I still get angry.

At other times Debbie's anger turns to helplessness and frustration.

> Even now I feel helpless when he's in such pain just getting out of bed and there's nothing I can do about it. It's awful seeing a person you don't care about in pain, so when it's someone close to you it's even more difficult.

These days Paul and Debbie find they cope best by not talking about arthritis.

> I know there's no going back. The damage to my joints has been done. There are no dreams that things could be better than they are. I have to make the most of the mobility I have. In a way I'm grateful because at least I can get around and I can earn my living.

'We acknowledge the arthritis is there,' says Debbie,

> but now I even ask him to come ballroom dancing with me. He can't twirl around like a mad thing the way some of them do but he tries and he enjoys it. Part of me knows it's not fair but I want him to be my partner not someone else.

Accepting the limitations your illness can inflict on you is even more difficult when your partner cannot accept them. Unlike Paul, Ann, a fifty-seven-year-old housewife, who has osteoarthritis and Crohn's disease, feels her husband of thirty-four years hasn't given her the understanding she's needed.

> My husband has said such cruel things over the years. He's even told me that if he'd known I'd become so ill he wouldn't have married me. He does love me, I know. He's just shut off his emotions

because I'm sure he can't bear the thought that anything will happen to me.

I'm not criticising my husband when I say these things because I can understand what he's having to cope with. Living with someone who's never going to get better is difficult for a healthy, active person. I've noticed that couples who knew about a partner's disability before they married sometimes cope so much better.

Ann strongly believes that her chronic illnesses have put a terrible strain on her marriage, particularly because of her husband's resentment and bitterness.

There's no spontaneity in our marriage now. We used to be such a lively, active couple – these days I can't go anywhere without planning. I've even had to have a loo put in downstairs because my osteoarthritis means I can't move very quickly. When you have Crohn's disease you have to go to the loo as soon as possible when you feel the need. Because of the stiffness in my joints – particularly my knees – I'd had several accidents on my slow climb up the stairs.

Another strain on our marriage comes from the sexual side. The spontaneity of sex and loving has totally gone. Even today people with disabilities don't talk openly about sexual problems. I find it very embarrassing to talk about it myself. Yet I find sex intolerable because of my ill-health and the pain and discomfort I'm in. So now it's non-existent. That makes me feel guilty about my husband's needs. I'm sure my marriage has been ruined because of illness. We get on but there's no sparkle.

Ann agrees that taking a positive attitude and coming to terms with arthritis are two of the best means of self-help.

But she finds that some people advise you to do this in such a glib and patronising way that it makes her really angry.

> I have accepted my life and I have a fuller life than before because of the other sufferers I've met and the joy I get from them when they've achieved something.
>
> Mike [she means me here!], who is my favourite medical broadcaster, is even guilty of making light of his advice. When I listen to him on the *Jimmy Young Show* I get so mad sometimes. I know he's right when he says you have to learn to adapt but it's much, much more difficult than a healthy person realises. Life can be good again but with a different set of ground rules.
>
> All this constant advice to adapt and to make the best of your situation makes you feel as if you are a wimp on the days when you just want to sit down and have a good cry.

Sorry, Ann. I'm just trying to help you as best I can in an imperfect world. But on your good days you agree that a positive attitude and acceptance of the illness are benefits. And no doubt this has helped you to find support and joy from sharing the successes of other sufferers – in spite of your husband's resentment of the restrictions to your life. There's certainly no shame in sitting down and having a good cry – you're not a wimp! – because crying releases the body's endorphins, those natural salves of pain, both physical and emotional. A good cry probably does as much good as a prescription. I know how irritating it must be to be constantly told that taking a positive attitude to arthritis can help, but believe me, being determined you're not going to let arthritis rule your life *is* important.

Talking to other people with arthritis can help some sufferers. Seeing how successfully one person is managing to cope with the disease can raise your expectations as well as offer you mutual support. There's no point waiting for the pain to disappear before you do something and try to enjoy life again. And don't turn your back on counselling, for example, if you've had an unhappy adolescence or suffer difficult family relationships or strains on your marriage because of your arthritis.

If you can't do something look at it as a challenge to try to find a way round it. And when you've found another way, think to yourself you've scored a point against arthritis and not given in to it. Feeling helpless just makes the disease itself seem worse.

Don't focus on the things you *can't* do but on the things you *can*. Negative thoughts just bring on more negative thoughts in my opinion and then you become trapped in a vicious circle of gloom. Many sufferers are convinced that the pain of arthritis is affected by their moods – when they're fed up they somehow feel the pain more. This makes you more stressed and depressed. Then once you're down, it becomes much harder to cope with everything, your arthritis included. So fighting pain, with painkillers and with your mind, is important.

COMPLEMENTARY OR ALTERNATIVE TREATMENTS

Some figures suggest that as many as a third of arthritis sufferers have tried complementary medicine. You may find this surprising but pain is a very subjective thing and if you've never known the constant pain arthritis can cause, it's easy to dismiss people's quest for pain relief.

Most practitioners of unconventional therapies prefer the use of the term 'complementary' medicine rather than 'alternative' because they feel their treatment should work side by side with more conventional methods. I'm in favour of their treatments whatever you call them – but do let both your doctor and the complementary practitioner know that you're seeking the help of both. And listen to their advice and their opinions on the value or the dangers. Your doctor is likely to suggest more of the former but it's important to ask.

Remember that these treatments may help relieve pain in some cases but I don't believe they can cure or stop the disease process. Also be aware that you don't have to have your doctor's approval to try these treatments, although, as I've said, I would suggest checking with him first to rule out any possibility of risk in your individual case.

ACUPUNCTURE

For many people the mention of acupuncture gives rise to thoughts of acting as a pin-cushion with needles being stuck here, there and everywhere. In reality, acupuncture has been an accepted form of treatment in China for around five thousand years and these days more and more people in the West are turning to it for a wide variety of ills. Many people believe it is extremely effective in easing a wide variety of conditions, by – in simple terms – stimulating the patient's own healing responses. Conditions that can benefit include headaches and migraine, skin problems, back pain, tinnitus, insomnia and even depression, as well as possibly arthritis.

I'm regularly asked what acupuncture involves and how it can help you. One theory is that it stimulates the brain to produce the chemicals endorphins – raised levels have been detected in tests twenty minutes after treatment. As I pointed out earlier, endorphins are the body's natural painkillers.

Traditional acupuncture is a 'holistic' form of medicine – a philosophy which not only treats the symptom but aims to improve the total well-being of the patient. Practitioners believe that many physical conditions can be worsened by, or be a result of, emotional stress, poor diet, and other factors. So your first visit to an acupuncturist will probably include detailed questions about your lifestyle and a thorough examination. The tongue is especially important in making a diagnosis so don't be surprised if this comes under careful scrutiny.

Acupuncture aims to correct any disharmony within the body – to achieve a balance between Yin and Yang. An imbalance, they say, can lead to disease. There are different traditions of acupuncture but they all revolve around the basic principle that the body has an intricate network of linking pathways, 'meridians', which carry our vital 'energies' through the body. These cannot be seen but can be detected using special techniques and can be likened to the nerve pathways known to Western doctors.

There are twelve main meridians either side of the body, each related to specific organs, such as the heart, liver and stomach. Twelve different pulses on the wrists also relate to the various organs and these are felt, and many other factors taken into account, when the traditional acupuncturist is deciding on treatment. Some practitioners – many GPs, for instance – have undertaken a short course in acupuncture (not involving the whole philosophy) and will use it in a limited way, for example, to relieve pain.

Each meridian has many points along it in precise positions called 'acupoints'. During acupuncture very fine needles are inserted into several of these points according to the problem being treated. So by inserting needles or by using pressure, the correct flow and balance of energies can be restored. The needles used are solid and finer than the type used for injections and you normally feel a slight prick when the needle is inserted into the skin.

This treatment may help to relieve pain in arthritis but it won't repair joint damage and may not be of any benefit during an active stage of rheumatoid arthritis. No one can predict who will respond, but one study in a general practice showed that 70 per cent of people complaining of various aches and pains in their muscles and bones were likely to be helped by acupuncture. And according to ARC, in one study osteoarthritis sufferers with painful swollen knees were given acupuncture while others tried hydrocortisone injections. Acupuncture was found to relieve the pain for a longer time though it didn't help the swelling. But pain relief for some people – long-lasting or not – is obviously more important than the precise scientific explanation of how acupuncture works.

To be on the safe side, ask your doctor's advice before deciding to try acupuncture for your symptoms. He or she may also be able to recommend a practitioner for you. Sometimes acupuncture can be used in conjunction with conventional medicine to improve the patient's general health.

Always be sure to go to a well-qualified acupuncturist – those with letters after their name such as BAAR or TAS, for example. Any adverse effects should then be most unlikely and you can be confident that the needles used will be properly sterilised. For addresses, see page 100.

HOMOEOPATHY

Homoeopathy is said to be a completely safe form of therapy and homoeopathic medicines are even available under the National Health Service.

This form of treatment is relatively new in comparison with acupuncture. It was first developed nearly two hundred years ago by a German physician, scholar and chemist, Samuel Hahnemann, out of the principle that 'like cures like'. Symptoms are treated by giving a minute dose of a substance which if given in larger quantities to a healthy person will actually cause those symptoms. Even in conventional medicine this principle is sometimes used – for instance, controlled doses of radiation are given to cure cancer, which can be *caused* by too much radiation.

Homoeopathists believe in the body's natural ability to heal itself. A homoeopath will therefore aim to give a remedy which will encourage this process of stimulating the body's natural forces of recovery – unlike a conventional doctor who prescribes medicines to suppress symptoms (aspirin, for instance, to bring down a temperature, or anti-histamines to dry up a runny nose).

Many homoeopaths are qualified doctors who have done a further year's training in homoeopathy. They may become GPs or work in homoeopathic hospitals (there are about six of these in the UK) and their treatment is available on the NHS, or they may consult privately. The advantage of consulting a medically qualified homoeopath is that they are trained in diagnosis. If you do consult a homoeopath who is not also a doctor, make sure he or she has done a full homoeopathic training at an approved college.

Obviously, homoeopathy isn't going to help, for example, the person with advanced osteoarthritis of the hip. But some people have found that it helps ease their pain and discomfort – and anything that can do that, in the hands of a responsible professional, must be good.

Both New Era and Weleda make a range of homoeopathic remedies which are widely available in health shops and even some chemists such as Boots. Those suggested for arthritis are *Apis mellifica, Arnica montana, Bryonia alba* and *Calcarea fluorica.*

OSTEOPATHY

Osteopathy began in the 1870s in the United States and it lays main emphasis on the structural and mechanical problems of the body. In other words the osteopath is most concerned with correcting faults in the musculo-skeletal system which is made up of the bones, joints, muscles, ligaments and connective tissue.

Osteopaths believe that many diseases are due to parts of the skeleton becoming misplaced and should consequently be treated by gentle methods of adjustment. They use a variety of techniques ranging from gentle massage or stretching movements to manipulation.

(As the law stands at the moment anyone in the United Kingdom can claim they are an osteopath so if you want to try this treatment make sure the osteopath has the title Registered Osteopath or the letters MRO after his or her name.)

Please remember that when your joints are actually damaged by arthritis, manipulation or massage can't undo that damage. I don't believe it can miraculously restore your joints to the way they were before disease set in, and you should certainly not undergo any form of manipulation if you're going through a flare-up or have any inflammation.

Reputable osteopaths won't claim they can cure your arthritis but they may be able to provide temporary pain relief. They wouldn't treat the inflammation as such and wouldn't treat you if you were in an acute phase of arthritis. They would also certainly question you to enable them to understand your medical background as well as your lifestyle.

Some rheumatoid arthritis sufferers find manipulation helpful. Given to the right patient in the right way, it can be helpful in the short-term but, regrettably, there is no evidence that it reverses the changes due to arthritis. It's important, too, to be sure that the practitioner has seen an x-ray of your joint, and so is fully aware of the extent of the condition, before manipulation commences.

CHIROPRACTIC

Chiropractic is a method of healing based on a manipulation of the spine and is not to be confused with chiropody – care of the feet. Surprisingly, it isn't especially well known despite being the third largest healing profession in the world, after medicine and dentistry.

Like osteopathic treatment, chiropractic has been known to bring relief when performed by the right hands to the right person. But if your joints are inflamed, as they can so often be in rheumatoid arthritis and in ankylosing spondylitis, manipulation can be damaging. A qualified practitioner will know that.

If you want to try this treatment contact the British Chiropractors' Association for a chiropractor in your area. To become a chiropractor, students must take a four-year, full-time course at a recognised college, leading to a BSc degree in Chiropractic, followed by a further year post-graduate course at an established clinic. Only then can an application be made for full membership of the British Chiropractic Association.

Another point to remember is that there's no average length for the course of treatment you may need. When a condition is diagnosed that cannot benefit from chiropractic, such as acute inflammatory disease or rheumatoid arthritis, your chiropractor will refer you elsewhere.

USEFUL ADDRESSES

ARC, Arthritis and Rheumatism Council for Research, Copeman House, St Mary's Court, St Mary's Gate, Chesterfield, Derbyshire S41 7TD. Tel: 0246 558033. The ARC is the only national charity in the UK raising money solely to further research into and knowledge of rheumatic disease. It relies entirely on voluntary contributions yet still manages to raise more than £10 million a year. It also produces many informative and helpful leaflets on all aspects of arthritis, in addition to a lively magazine called *Arthritis Research Today*.

Arthritis Care, 18 Stephenson Way, London NW1 2HD. Tel: 071 916 1500. Arthritis Care is a national voluntary organisation which provides information, advice and help by letter and phone (either on the main number or on the helpline 0800 289170, calls free of charge on weekday afternoons). It campaigns for greater public awareness of the needs and problems associated with arthritis. It runs specially equipped holiday centres, self-catering holiday units and a residential home for those who are very disabled. It also provides regular meetings of more than five hundred local branches.

Young Arthritis Care is a section of Arthritis Care and is a self-help support group run by and for all young people with arthritis – anybody up to the age of forty-five. There are more than fifty nationwide contacts who are either young people with arthritis or parents of children with arthritis who help, support and advise others in similar situations to their own.

There are local groups around the country that allow members to get together, share information and give each other advice and support. Young Arthritis Care would love to hear from you if you would be interested in being a contact.

The group also prints a magazine, runs personal development courses and organises holidays for children and teenagers.

The Arthritic Association, Hill House, 1 Little New Street, London EC4A 3TR. Tel: 071 491 0233. The association was founded in 1942 in Bournemouth by a group of forty-nine people who had overcome symptoms of arthritis. It's now a registered charity (number 292569) which encourages the use of 'natural'

methods of treating arthritis. These include homoeopathic remedies, sensible eating and in some cases massage therapy.

The Association for Swimming Therapy, c/o Ted Cowan, 4 Oak
Street, Shrewsbury SY3 7RH. Tel: 0743 344393. Swimming for
people with disabilities. About two hundred clubs are affiliated to
the association – contact them to find out if there's one near you.

The British Homoeopathic Association, 27a Devonshire Street,
London W1N 1RJ. Tel: 071 935 2163. For books, advice, information and a list of practitioners.

The Chartered Society of Physiotherapy, 14 Bedford Row,
London WC1R 4ED. Tel: 071 242 1941. For further information
on physiotherapy and also private practice physiotherapists.

College of Occupational Therapists, 6–8 Marshalsea Road,
Southwark, London SE1 1HL. Tel: 071 357 6480. You can contact
the college for information on a private practice register.

The Council for Acupuncture, 179 Gloucester Place, London
NW1 6DX. Tel: 071 724 5756. Send £2 and a large s.a.e. for a
directory of British acupuncturists.

Dial Disablement – a local information and advice line. The DIAL
service can provide information about local services including the
possibility of local suppliers who loan or sell equipment. Look
under the 'Disabled – amenities and information' section in your
phone directory for such a service in your area.

Disabled Living Foundation, 380–4 Harrow Road, London SW9
2HU. Tel: 071 289 6111. The foundation is a national charity and
provides practical advice and information in particular on equipment for disabled people and their carers. It runs an equipment
centre in London for people to view (open from 9–5, Mondays to
Fridays). Viewing is by appointment and many find that an
appointment with one of the centre's staff is extremely helpful.
The centre isn't a shop but offers impartial advice on equipment
on the market. Contact the foundation by letter or by ringing the
above number and ask for the Information Service.

General Council and Register of Osteopaths, 56 London Street,
Reading, Berkshire RG1 4SQ. Tel: 0734 576585 for names and
addresses of registered osteopaths in your area.

Lupus UK, Queens Court, 9–17 Eastern Road, Romford, Essex
RN1 3NG. Tel: 0708 731251. A charity operating self-help groups
throughout the UK for people with lupus. It provides advice and
counselling on all aspects of the disease and publishes national and
regional newsletters as well as raising funds for research.

NACC, National Association for Colitis and Crohn's Disease, 98A London Road, St Albans, Herts AL1 1NX. Tel: 0727 44296. Information and support for inflammatory bowel disease sufferers – a small percentage of whom develop arthritis as a consequence of the disease.

National Ankylosing Spondylitis Society, 5 Grosvenor Crescent, London SW1X 7ER. Tel: 071 235 9585. The society has around sixty groups throughout the country usually meeting one evening a week in a hospital for group physiotherapy. It also provides book lists, publications, a cassette of a twenty-minute programme of physiotherapy exercises, as well as producing a twice-yearly newsletter containing articles by doctors and sufferers on different aspects of the disease.

The National Institute of Medical Herbalists, 9 Palace Gate, Exeter EX1 1JA. Tel: 0392 426022.

The Psoriasis Association, 7 Milton Street, Northampton NN2 7JG. Tel: 0604 711129. The association is a self-help group providing social contact, advice and collecting funds for and promoting research.

RADAR Royal Association for Disability and Rehabilitation, 25 Mortimer Street, London W1N 8AB. Tel: 071 637 5400. This organisation campaigns for, among other things, the removal of barriers to disabled people be it architectural, economic or just people's attitudes. You can ring its general advice line for information on entitlement to services, aid and equipment or housing, for example. Call the above number and ask for the information department.

Royal College of Surgeons, 35–43 Lincoln's Inn Fields, London WC2A 3PN. Tel: 071 405 3474. Contact the college for leaflets aimed at the public, explaining common operations.

The government's patient Charter has resulted in the setting up of Regional Health Information Services to provide information about waiting lists (extremely useful if you are awaiting joint replacement surgery), NHS services, self-help groups and common illnesses.

East Anglia, East Anglian Healthlink. Tel: 0345 678 333.

Mersey, Healthwise. Tel: 0800 838 909.

North East Thames, Health Information Service (managed by College of Health). Tel: 0345 678 444.

North Western, Patients' Advice Bureau. Tel: 0345 678 888.

North West Thames, Health Information Service. Tel: 0345 678 400.
Northern, Health Info North. Tel: 0345 678 100.
Oxford, Health Info Line. Tel: 0345 678 700.
Pan Thames, Waiting List Helpline. Tel: 0345 678 150.
South East Thames, Health Directory. Tel: 0345 678 500.
South Western, Open Health. Tel: 0345 678 777.
South West Thames, SW Thames Health Information.
Tel: 0345 678 555.
Trent, Trent Healthline. Tel: 0345 678 300.
Wessex, Wessex Health Information (managed by the charity Heal for Health Trust). Tel: 0345 678 679.
West Midlands, Midlands Health Point. Tel: 0345 678 800.
Yorkshire, Healthbox. Tel: 0345 678 200.

In addition to these regional health information services there's also an independent charity called the **Help for Health Trust** (Tel: 0962 849100). It was established by Wessex Regional Health Authority and provides information to the people of Hampshire, Isle of Wight, Dorset, Wiltshire and the Bath area. The Trust says it helps people to become active partners in their own health care by providing them with the information they need to make healthy choices.

AUSTRALIA

The Arthritis Foundation of Australia, National Office, Suite 421, Wingello House, Angel Place, Sydney 2000, Australia, Tel: 02-221-2456

Funds research on arthritis and other rheumatic diseases. Has affiliated organisations all over Australia for arthritis sufferers.

The Australian Association of Occupational Therapists Inc, 6 Spring Street, Fitzroy, Victoria 3065, Australia, Tel: 03-416-1021

Australian Crohn's and Colitis Association, PO Box 201, Mooroolbark, Victoria 3138, Australia

South Australian Crohn's and Colitis Association Inc, PO Box 3153, Grenfell Street, Adelaide SA 500, Australia

Lupus Association of NSW Inc, PO Box 89, North Ryde 2113, Australia, Tel: 878 6055

Victorian Lupus Assoc Inc, PO Box 811F, GPO Melbourne 3001

The Lupus/Scleroderma Group, The Arthritis Foundation of Australia-SA, 99 Anzac Highway, Ashford 5035, Tel: 297 2488

CANADA

The Arthritis Society, 250 Bloor Street East, Suite 401, Toronto, Ontario M4W 3P2, Tel: 416-967-1414

Mr Lorne Ferley, Manitoba Ankylosing Spondylitis Association, 19 Carolyn Bay, Winnipeg, Manitoba R2J 2Z3, Canada, Tel: 204-256-5320

Ankylosing Spondylitis Association of British Colombia, c/o Arthritis Society, 895 W10th Avenue, Vancouver, British Colombia V55 1L7, Tel: 879-7511

Mr Nils Linholm, Ontario Spondylitis Association, 250 Bloor St East, Suite 401, Toronto, Ontario M4W 3P2, Tel: 416-967-1414

The Canadian Association of Occupational Therapists, 110 Eglinton Avenue West, 3rd Floor, Toronto, Ontario M4R 1A3, Canada, Tel: 416-487-5404

Canadian Foundation for Ileitis and Colitis, 21 St Clair Avenue East, Suite 301, Toronto, Ontario, Canada M4T 1L9

or
PO Box 5652, Station B, Victoria, British Colombia V8R 6S4, Canada

Lupus Canada, Box 3302, Station B, Clagary, Alberta T2M 418, Tel: 1-800-661-1468

INDEX

ankylosing spondylitis 18–24, 40, 45:
    age 18, 19, anaemia 21; case
    histories 19–21, 22–4; colitis,
    Crohn's disease 30; depression
    24–5; drugs 20–21, 22; ESR test
    21–2; exercise 22; eyesight 21;
    genetic factor 19–20;
    inflammation 18–19, 98; male/
    female incidence 19; misdiagnosis
    19–20; morning stiffness 18; sex,
    relationships 23; surgery 22;
    symptoms 18, 22, 30
American National Institute of Health
    78
anterior uveitis 21
Arthritic Association 74–5
Arthritis & Rheumatism Council
    (ARC) 45, 72, 79–80, 81, 95
Arthritis Care 13, 64
Association for Swimming Therapy
    60

Bouchard's nodes 9
British Chiropractic Association 98
British Medical Journal 52

carpal tunnel syndrome 3
Chartered Society of Physiotherapy
    58
chiropractic 20, 98
cold treatments 69–70
colitic arthritis 18
collagen diseases 38–9
College of Occupational Therapists 64
Crohn's disease, arthritis and 28–33,
    89–90: age 29; case history
    30–33; depression 31; drugs 33;
    enteropathic arthritis 29–30;
    morning stiffness 30–31; other
    sufferers 31–2, 91; sex/marriage
    90; surgery 33; symptoms 29; *see
    also* ulcerative colitis

dermatomyositis 39
diet and supplements 5, 70–81: alcohol
    72, 77; balanced 70, 76, 78; case
    histories 73–7; evening primrose
    oil 72, 76, 81; fish-oil
    supplements 72–4, 76, 79; green-
    lipped mussel extract 79–80;
    herbal remedies 80–81; low-fat

74; oily fish 72–4; propolis 74;
    royal jelly 80; selenium 73, 79;
    weight 78–9; wholefood 75
drugs 37, 41, 43, 49–50: anti-
    inflammatory 20–21, 49–50, 59,
    74–5, 86; anti-rheumatic 49–50;
    gold-based 50, 86; immuno-
    suppressives 41, 50; painkillers
    49, 68–9; steroids 41, 43, 45–6,
    50, 59, 75
Disabled Living Foundation 64

endorphins 56, 83, 91, 94
enteropathic arthritis 29–30
erthrocyte sedimentation rate (ESR)
    test 21–2, 46
exercise 22, 55, 57–8, 82–4: aerobics
    83; contact sport 17, 82–3; pain
    82; rest 82–3; stress 82–3;
    swimming 82; walking 82–3

German measles (rubella) 3
gout 33–8, 49, 71: age 35; blood test
    diagnosis 35; case history 35–7;
    cause 34; crystal deposits (tophi)
    34–5, 37; deformity 35; diet 36–8,
    71–2; drugs 37–8, 49; enzyme
    defect 37; genetic factor 37; male/
    female incidence 35, 37;
    menopause 37; purines 34, 37,
    72; symptoms 34; uric acid 34–7,
    49, 72; weight 37, 38

Hahnemann, Samuel 96
Health Education Authority 82
heat treatment 69–70
Heberden's nodes 9
homoeopathy 20, 96–7: remedies 75,
    96–7

immune system 11, 13, 29, 38, 45, 50,
    52, 71, 79
iritis 21

joint replacement 45, 51, 78–9: hip 22,
    26–8, 51–4; knee 8, 13, 54;
    shoulder 13

Lupus UK 40

National Ankylosing Spondylitis
    Society (NASS) 19, 22, 23

National Association for Colitis and Crohn's disease (NACC) 29
National Institute of Medical Herbalists 81

occupational therapy 42, 46, 55, 60–68: aids, equipment 61–6; energy preservation 63; 'joint preservation' 61–2, 82; management 61, 63; pain reduction 61

osteoarthritis 3, 4, 11, 15, 29, 53, 89: age 4–6, 8, 12; acupuncture 95–6; bending aids 63–4; case history 6–8; development of 8–9; genetic factor 5, 10; injury 9–10; joint disfigurement 8–9; menopause 10; misdiagnosis 6; monarticular 9; remission 78; symptoms 9, 11; surgery 78–9; wear and tear 5, 8; weight 10, 78–9; weight-bearing joints 9, 12

osteoarthritis see osteoarthritis
osteopathy 20, 97–8

physiotherapy 10, 46, 52, 55–60, 82: exercises 55, 57–8; Faradic footbaths 56–7; hydrotheraphy 58–60; infra-red 56–7; interferential therapy 55–6; laser 56; oxygen 56; splinting 60; traction 56; transcutaneous nerve stimulator (TENS) 56–7; ultrasonic 56; use of joints 58

polyartheritis nodosa 3, 39
polymyositis 39
positive thinking 85–92: attitude of partners 86–90, 92; case histories 85–91; confidence 86–7; counselling 92

psoriatic arthritis 18, 24–33: case history 25–8; depression 27; fatigue 25; fellow-sufferers 27–8; morning stiffness 25; sex life 28; surgery 26–7; symptoms 24–5, 26

psoriasis 24–8: age 24; stress 27–8; symptoms 24, 26

reactive arthritis 3, 18
reflexology 20
Reiter's syndrome 3, 18, 85
relaxation 68, 82, 84–5

rheumatoid arthritis 4–5, 7, 9, 10–18, 19, 24, 29, 38, 39, 41, 42, 44–5, 59, 65: acupuncture 95; age 10, 12; case histories 14–18, 73–7; copper bracelets 81; damage by 11; development of 10–11; diet 73–7; disablement 10–11, 13, 16; drugs 50, 59; eyes 12; genetic factor 11; hands, tendons of 11, 14; immune system 11, 12; inflammatory nature 10–12, 98; large joints 12; male/female incidence 12; misdiagnosis 16; morning stiffness 13, 14, 66; muscle wasting 14; osteopathy 97–8; remission 13, 78; small joints 12; symptoms 12–13; synovial membrane 11

rheumatoid factor test 47
rubs and liniments 70

scleroderma 13, 38
septic arthritis 38
seronegative spondarthropathies 18
Sjogren's syndrome 13
spiritual healing 43–4
Sports Council 82
surgery 51–4, 65: knee, condylor joints 54, synovectomy 51, 86; hip (arthroplasty) 51–4; shoulder 13, 54; ulnar drift 51

synovial membrane 11, 14
systemic lupus erythematosus 13, 38–44, 50: age 39; anaemia 39; anti-body test 39–40; case history 41–4; drugs 4, 41, 43; fatigue 39, 41, 43, 83; genetic factor 40; immune system 38–9; male/female incidence 39–40; menstruation 40; misdiagnosis 40; oral ulcers 39; photosensitivity 40, 42; pregnancy 39–40; symptoms 39–41

systemic sclerosis see scleroderma

treatment 45–67: see drugs; occupational therapy; physiotherapy; self-help; surgery

ulcerative colitis, arthritis and 28–30: age 29; stress 29